OUT WITH THE OLD

ENJOYING THE TRIP TO AGE 120

Tricia Keene, Ph.D.

RSE Publishing
Laurens, South Carolina

First Printing June 2012

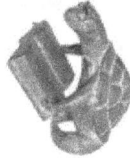

Printed in the United States of America
Book Design by Michael Seymour

Table of Contents

Chapter One:
*Introduction, Expectations, and
Vision for 120*
1

Chapter Two:
Aging in an Exceptional Fashion
17

Chapter Three:
Leadership Development in Midlife
25

Chapter Four:
Step One: Positioning for Change
31

Chapter Five:
Step Two: Self-discovery
41

Chapter Six:
Intellectual Stimulation
53

Chapter Seven:
Physical Well Being
57

Chapter Eight:
Social Networking
67

Chapter Nine:
Emotional Literacy
71

Chapter Ten:
Spiritual Growth
81

Chapter Eleven:
*Step Three: A Broader, Deeper
Sense of Purpose*

89

Chapter Twelve:
Step Four: Pursuit of Unique Potential

97

Summary and Conclusion

117

"AGE IS A QUESTION OF MIND OVER MATTER.

IF YOU DON'T MIND, IT DOESN'T MATTER."

LEROY "SATCHEL" PAIGE

Acknowledgements

I am grateful for the many teachers and business associates who have entered my life to hone my functional, educational, and business skills over the years. Yet, it is those outside the institutional and corporate walls who have shaped my personal growth in unforeseeable ways:

My parents, who modeled through their own lives a standard of unconditional love.

My siblings, who are cherished for our common backgrounds and histories over time.

Warren, who has grown with me as we've faced "the good, the bad, and the ugly" during our 39 years of marriage.

Tim, Jeff, and Deanna, who have truly made my life worthwhile.

Joe Gauld and the faculty, administration, parents, and students at the Hyde School, who inspired me to take a deeper look at myself.

Tom McNeil and John Decker at TMI Executive Resources who took me on an invaluable journey inside life transitions.

Dr. Pat Ward-Baker, who helped keep our collective passion for enriching longevity alive.

My many NYNEX co-workers and friends, both lifelong and new, who continue to challenge my personal growth through their own experiences and ongoing learning.

The Osher Lifelong Learning Institute (OLLI) which continues to inspire so many of us to pursue new learning opportunties.

The Cliffs staff and Dr. Holbrook Raynal in South Carolina who have proven to be valuable "Wellness" resources.

Amanda Capps, my editor, who creatively helped me leapfrog ahead when my thoughts truncated in cul-de-sacs of sorts.

Sue Heiferman and John Asaro, my Cliffs photographers; and Dan Fowler, who contributed illustrations, for their efforts on the finishing touches of this book.

1

INTRODUCTION, EXPECTATIONS, AND VISION FOR 120

"LIFE BEFORE SIXTY IS NOTHING BUT A WARM-UP."
BILL HINSON

Introduction

Evolving research on longevity makes it clear that living to 100 is no longer an anomaly, but entirely possible. A recent article in *The Wall Street Journal* stated that one in four of today's sixty-five-year-olds will live to age ninety in the United States. According to the Census Bureau, the number of Americans age sixty-five and older has grown 15.1 percent to 40.3 million since 2000, faster than the United States population which grew 9.7 percent. Of the "oldest old" (85-100 plus), the 90-94 year olds had the greatest increase in percentage growth. In fact, living to 120 is now a possibility for some of us. With modern science working in our favor, as well as the adoption of the common sense principles in this book, you could be one of those lucky, amazing people still swinging at 120!

With that in mind, it is clear that our view of the 100-120-year-old person in our minds needs a drastic revision. None of us wishes to live out our later years alone in sickness and depression. With a new vision of the healthy, energetic, alert, and engaging person you'll be at 120, we can chart the course from where you are now to where you'll want to be then. I, for one, am not willing to give up.

Frankly, neither the concept nor the practice of "retirement" has worked well for me. My first retirement at age forty-nine didn't last long. After twenty-seven years in telecommunications, I took only a two-week respite before diving back into the working world as vice president of an energy services firm. The latter was a 150-year-old firm, and I became the first female to hold an executive operations assignment there. Being first was not new to me; I had been the first female at NYNEX to hold an executive operations position with responsibility for 9,600 employees in two companies. In the earlier years of my career, I was often the first female to work in a number of field operations positions. Back in 1977, I undoubtedly was the first female to have my water break in the dining hall at the AT&T headquarters in Basking Ridge, New Jersey. That was my first experience with childbirth. Fortunately, my other two children were kind enough to start the labor process in a more private, domestic environment.

My retirement from energy services lasted all of six months as I sifted through various opportunities. I decided to start my own consulting firm focused on measurements but quickly realized that there was little new growth in that for me. Indeed, it felt as though I was turning back the clock ten years. That is when it dawned on me that what I really wanted to do was return to school to pursue a Ph.D. in leadership development. I had always valued education and had already earned a bachelor's degree in mathematics from the University of Maine and an MBA from the Whittemore School of Business and Economics at the University of New Hampshire. The doctoral work, however, would be pivotal, as revelations I had during that time led to my writing this book. In order to fulfill a requirement of my Ph.D. program, I sought an internship at a firm at which I later became a senior vice president. My job involved counseling middle managers and executives worldwide who were making major transitions in their lives. I felt I was a seasoned veteran of positive transitions, and while working in that capacity, I began to note some common characteristics of people who moved from one phase of life to another with purpose and vigor.

My third retirement from that position came six years later. Our three children had finished college, and my husband and I were considering a move. Ultimately, we chose a picturesque mountain community in Upstate South Carolina. With this retirement, however, I still had no plans to stop working or growing. As an incessant learner focused on enriching longevity, I was struck by the numbers of extremely talented retired young (in my terms) people in the area who had essentially put their leadership skills on the shelf without giving thought to a new sense of purpose. And thus began my next career. For the last seven years, I have been working with people in their midlife years from their forties through their nineties. Together, we create new positive personal visions with a roadmap of how to get there. It is a passion from which I am not likely to retire . . . ever! If you are one of these people intent on living an extraordinary life up to age 100 or 120, read on and grow.

Shall We Live?

Each time I begin a seminar on living to age 120, some of the attendees question the wisdom of one who would even WANT to live that long. That is where it is perhaps illuminating to take a look at some facts. Simply put, many of us are in this life for the long haul–whether we like it or not. From my point of view, if I'm taking the ride no matter what, I'm going to enjoy the trip.

Although it may be difficult to ensure that the 2010 centenarian (people age one hundred and older) census figures are totally accurate due to birth record errors and access to that population, the Census Bureau reflects a population of 53,364. However, the 65 and over age group is expected to grow rapidly over the next decade with the wave of Baby Boomers. By 2050, the population of centenarians could approach one million. I'll be 105 in 2050 and plan to be counted among the million. I never thought I'd make it to the year 2000, which seemed four lifetimes away during my teenage years. You can calculate what age you will be in 2050, and make your own decision as to whether you want to be among the one million still in the game, but I suggest you delay that decision until after you finish this book. And by the way, your decision alone will make a difference.

Of note is the fact that the United States has the highest number of centenarians in the world, followed by Japan, which has a centenarian population about half that of the United States. On his or her 100th birthday, a Japanese centenarian receives a certificate and a silver sake chalice from the prime minister to signify longevity and prosperity. The diameter of the chalice was reduced as the centenarian population grew and the government suffered financial pressures.

In the United States, there has been a tradition that the President would send a letter to new centenarians, and since 1983, NBC's "Today Show" has announced known names. Other countries such as Italy, England, Ireland, and Sweden also honor centenarians in some fashion. It appears age is still noted–and sometimes revered in our society; however, I believe we have some ground to cover in terms of a complete image upgrade for the modern "senior." The time has come for today's vital representatives of the over-sixty set to be recognized for their crucial contributions–and I'm not talking about contributions in the past tense. Years ago, we acknowledged that forty was the new thirty. In the early decades of the twenty-first century, we must acknowledge and appreciate the fact that we live in a world with seventy-year-olds whose greatest work and happiest days could still be ahead of them.

With a growing number of centenarians, it is also interesting to look at the demographics of this amazing group. *The North American Actuarial Journal* uses Medicare records to make its estimates; it claims that in 2006, 85.9 percent of centenarians were women. According to the 2010 Census Briefs, however, there has been a "pronounced growth in the male population 65 years and older, leading to a narrowing gap between males and females at the older ages."

As more folks reach one hundred, it makes sense that many of us will live beyond that milestone. The new word coined by researchers for those over 110 is "supercentenarians."

Let's Assume You Live . . .

Out with the Old has been a work in progress for some nine years. The idea was conceived in collaboration with a fellow student from my Ph.D. program. At the time, Dr. Pat Ward-Baker was a senior vice president at Morgan Stanley. She earned a Ph.D. focused on gerontology and was specifically interested in studying exceptional older people and their characteristics. I was interested in studying midlife leadership. It seemed natural to marry the two research efforts. After two joint ventures, I opted to continue to modify and update the material, taking the "show on the road." Since then, I have taught in a number of academic, community, and church settings. Additional joint ventures with Pat are in the planning stage.

The objective of the material is two-fold. We will create a new vision for your centenarian years that replaces the image of "old and unable" with one of someone who continues to be engaged in and contributing to society. This is not just cutesy verbiage or a naïve commentary on positive thinking. The world is different, and perhaps our mindsets should be as well. This book will help you prepare for that shift.

> THIS IS NOT JUST CUTESY VERBIAGE
> OR A NAÏVE COMMENTARY
> ON POSITIVE THINKING.

Our process will be a combination of theory and practice. The theory is intended to give credibility to the concepts by referring to works and research by the experts in relevant fields. These detours into academia also help me justify why I earned a Ph.D. in the first place. Frankly, my husband claims that the initials stand for "Piled Higher and Deeper." Perhaps so, but in a positive way. It is important to recognize the scholars who went before us on whose shoulders we stand, all of whom contribute to the growing body of knowledge on a subject.

On the other hand, the "practice" will allow me to share anecdotes that bring the theories to life. These will undoubtedly call to mind your own life experiences. Theories require real life experiences in order to illustrate usefulness. Then too, "practice" often introduces an element of humor. Don't forget that one of the ways to make this "ride" enjoyable is to laugh at ourselves along the way—starting now.

Laugh Lines

Two older women were discussing their husbands over lunch. "I do wish that my John would stop biting his nails. He makes me terribly nervous." "My Fred used to do the same thing," the other woman replied, "but I broke him of the habit." "Really, how?" asked the first woman. "Easy, I hid his teeth."

---

*The author of this classic joke and authors of all "Laugh Lines" in this book are unknown.

Stereotypes Happen

We begin to shape our view of "old age" at a very young age. Think back to some of the fairy tales you heard as a child. Hansel and Gretel, Snow White, and others had an ugly old witch as one of the main characters. Feeding off those images, I remember at a very young age being afraid of an old man who lived in our neighborhood, believing that his cane hid a sword or rifle he would use to slay young children. None of the children in the neighborhood would go to his door at Halloween; we thought he would probably hand out apples with razors in them. We even crossed the street when we saw him ambling our way on his walks. Children will be children, but how sad it is that these relatively harmless misgivings mature into rampant misconceptions about the intentions and abilities of older people.

As we continue to age, we hear people deny being any older than twenty-nine or maybe thirty-nine . . . ever. By age 48-52, most women have begun to enter the mysterious world of menopause, while men have their own midlife crises of sorts (witness my husband's purchase of the convertible sports car). The good news for women is that menopause is followed by "post menopausal zest," according to Dr. Christiane Lorthrop, author of *The Wisdom of Menopause*. I choose to believe Dr. Lothrop and to think that bliss will last another 45-55 years. I'm not sure what the male equivalent might be, but I do know that my sample of one, my husband, is a hiking machine at seventy years of age. I call that zest!

Beyond what our bodies are telling us, our government, retailers, and other organizations send us messages that give us pause to think that life is closing in on us. For example, at age:

- **Forty**–the Age Discrimination in Employment Act (ADEA) kicks in. Why would anyone discriminate against a forty-year-old?
- **Forty-ish**–we women begin to get advice from our hairdressers, who say that it is time to cut our hair

short to "look our age," and men's barbers begin to inch the sideburns a bit shorter. Shouldn't a hairstyle or cut be based on what is flattering to an individual?

- **Fifty to fifty-five**–we receive our AARP "invitation." Couldn't they wait a bit longer?
- **Sixty**–we become eligible for "senior discounts" at retail operations and the movies. Some grocery stores also give us a break; I love the fact that I get five percent off my grocery bill at Harris Teeter as a "senior" on Thursdays–ditto Publix on Wednesdays. However, I was a little taken aback last week when the young whipper-snapper cashier gave me the discount without my asking for it!
- **Sixty-two-ish**–we are eligible for Social Security and early retirement–at least for the moment.
- **Sixty-five**–the traditional age for full retirement (The Social Security Act). For those of us born after 1938, it's 65-67.
- **Seventy**–mandatory retirement for some professions.
- **Seventy and a half**–the age at which we must begin to take money out of our IRAs, should we be lucky enough to have any money left.

Clearly, some of the above are nice perks, and although I resent being seen as an elder who needs help, I'm definitely looking for my 10 percent off that cup of coffee at Dunkin' Donuts. Even the Transportation Security Administration is getting into the act with a recently announced trial at four airports that will allow passengers over seventy-five to keep their shoes and light jackets on when going through security. Apparently those over seventy-five pose less of a security risk. With that said, perhaps the biggest perk we get in these turbulent times is that we would most likely be the first to get released in a hostage situation.

And So It Ends . . .

Just ten short years ago, I was startled to find that most of the available literature on aging and growth didn't apply to those beyond age sixty-five. Rather, post-retirement publications harped on dependence, illness, and disability. A few sassy "Maxine-type" authors such as John Wagner joked bitterly about aging. Nonfiction writers were prolific in their dry diatribes on estate planning and money management for the mature adult. This is not to say that Maxine isn't funny or that living wills should never be discussed. My beef is more about what's not on the shelves, as opposed to what is. Should we assume from a trip to the bookstore or a search on Amazon that "it's all downhill from here"? I know enough atypical "seniors" to say with all certainty that there is an interest in continuing to look at leadership, values, self-improvement, and transitions in careers and relationships well after one "retires" once or twice.

I KNOW ENOUGH ATYPICAL "SENIORS" TO SAY WITH ALL CERTAINTY THAT THERE IS AN INTEREST IN CONTINUING TO LOOK AT LEADERSHIP, VALUES, SELF-IMPROVEMENT, AND TRANSITIONS IN CAREERS AND RELATIONSHIPS WELL AFTER ONE "RETIRES" ONCE OR TWICE.

Let's throw out those old limitations and craft a new vision and path for ourselves.

Alternative Images of "Old Age"

Researchers from Ohio State University probed the concept of old age and the point at which someone supposedly attains it. They determined that aging is a "highly individual experience." Really?

However, they went on to say that changes typically occur in our senses during certain decades of life: hearing, mid-forties; vision, touch, and taste in the mid-fifties; and smell, mid-seventies.

Perhaps the study needs to be expanded, or maybe I am an unusual case, but my husband claims that I have had selective hearing since my thirties. I know that my vision has been impaired since my early teens when I got my first pair of glasses. A footnote to that comment, however, is that last month's cataract surgery has restored my sight to between 20/20 and 20/25. It is no small miracle that I can see with the naked eye for the first time in fifty-three years.

Thankfully, my sense of taste has never wavered, especially as it relates to chocolate. Not being able to taste my homemade chocolate sauce would certainly be a heavy blow to my system.

With that said, Ohio State's last two research areas on smell and touch may ring true for me. My sense of smell has definitely changed from earlier years, although I am still south of seventy by four years. It is a gift that for some reason I have retained the ability to pick up good smells, such as muffins cooking in the oven or wood burning in a fireplace, right away. Yet, unpleasant odors, all of which will go unmentioned, I miss entirely, and this suits me just fine.

The sense of touch is another issue altogether. I cannot say when I lost it, but my sense of touch probably changed in my fifties, as suggested by Ohio State's research. Two recent incidents have convinced me that my touch is permanently altered. That is to say, I have lost my fingerprints and am left with smooth fingertips. On my laptop, I have the technical ability to sign in with my fingerprint, if only it would recognize my fingerprint. In addition, when applying for a "permit to carry" two years ago, I found that my fingerprints were rejected three times (the limit at which time they issue the permit with or without fingerprints). I guess this is not all bad, because I obviously won't be accused of crimes due to a trail of fingerprints.

Annoying though, is that I have great difficulty opening those plastic produce bags at the grocery store with my shiny fingers! The other day, I was struggling with that task, and the man standing next to me handed me his bag, which he had already opened. I thanked him, gladly accepting the bag, and threw my bananas into it. That's when he told me his secret: he spits on his fingers. Trying to be the polite person I am most of the time, I put the bag into my cart, hoping that the bananas were thick skinned.

The bottom line for me is that the Ohio State study had it right when the researchers allowed that aging is a "highly individual experience"!

The Age of Wisdom

Stephen Covey looked at aging on a broader scale and wrote about what he calls "The Five Ages of Civilization's Voice." He sifted through the ages over time, beginning with the hunter-gatherer, symbolized by a bow and arrow. Looking at the ages that followed, he brings us into today's world as the "Age of Wisdom," symbolized by a compass.

The compass signifies the power to choose our direction and purpose and to obey natural laws or principles (like magnetic north) that never change and are "universal, timeless, and self evident." Covey believes that deep within each of us, there is an inner longing to live a life of greatness and contribution, and that you and I have the potential to do so. I agree.

We can translate that to mean that every day when we get up, we can choose to have a good attitude about the day or a bad one. My husband can tell you that I often start my day singing, "Today is Tuesday (or Wednesday or whatever); you know what that means: it's going to be a special day . . ." Some of you will recall the lyrics from *The Mickey Mouse Club*, back in a time when people seemed a whole lot more optimistic than they do today.

Another interpretation of Covey's Age of Wisdom reflects a world in which we simply do and say what we're thinking, feeling, or are subconsciously driven to do and we do so with more regularity and comfort as we age, with less regard for what people think of us, thus bestowing a new sense of individual freedom. That freedom allows us to create a new vision for ourselves at age 120.

Creating A New Vision

Helen Keller once remarked, "Worse than not having sight is having no vision." There is an easy way to test the power of visioning. Try this exercise when you are alone somewhere. Lengthen your arms in front of you and grasp and point your fingers in front of you. Close your eyes. Move your fingertips and straight arms around to the right as far as you can possibly go. Take your time. Open your eyes and notice where your fingers are pointing. Notice how far you turned, as well as what is beyond that point.

Now start the exercise again. Point your arms and fingers as before, and close your eyes. This time, move around to the right further than you went before, remembering that further point you had seen. Once again, go as far as you possibly can. Now, open your eyes, and notice how far you turned this time. To a person, in groups for which we have done this exercise, people are able to turn further once they have a vision of the potential planted in their minds.

Given that, you might also take a minute or two to think of yourself at your 120th birthday party (and, yes, we will still party then). This is best done with your eyes closed in a quiet, comfortable setting while you breathe deeply and let yourself go. Think about where you are, who is with you, what you're wearing, what you're feeling, what you're doing . . . and just stay with it for a few minutes.

I do wish I could find out what you all saw; alas, I will have to rely on input from those who have gone before you. Generally, the mere suggestion of a party at that age allows folks to consider having fun and helps them see the possibility. If that was so for you, you are already well on your way to 120! If, on the other hand, you saw an image of yourself that was not what you would consider to be your best, so to speak, please accept that you just need more time to move to the positive.

My own 120th birthday party is an exciting one for me. I am looking quite spiffy in my new yoga pants and bright blue top. I am surrounded by my husband, children, grandchildren, great grandchildren, sister, brother, sisters-in-law, other relatives, and friends and neighbors of all ages from up and down the East Coast and Texas. The party is being held outside on a lovely June day, and I am no longer worried about my hair "falling." There is a feast spread out before us, along with a variety of drinks. However, my eyes are focused on the huge chocolate cake that resembles a wedding cake in the middle of a round table. Those over twenty-one are preparing a toast with red wine, and I too am sipping from a beautiful large chalice. The music is loud and wonderful. I look forward to getting out on the dance floor; that is, after my first piece of cake. I am enjoying the hugs all around and feel very loved, grateful, and proud. I am already thinking about what I'll do for my 130th–my vision must once again extend further.

2

AGING IN AN EXCEPTIONAL FASHION

"AGING SEEMS TO BE THE ONLY AVAILABLE
WAY TO LIVE A LONG LIFE."
KITTY O'NEILL COLLINS

Starting with the End

Let's start with the end in mind. In the Bible, Genesis 6:3, the Lord said, "My spirit will not contend with man forever, for he is mortal; his days will be a hundred and twenty." Clearly, living to 120 is not a new idea!

With that said, we all know that people of all ages can have negative impressions or assumptions about old age. I heard a story the other day about an incident in a hospital that illustrates this concept.

Hospital regulations require a wheelchair for patients who are being discharged. One student nurse found an elderly gentleman already dressed and sitting on the bed with a suitcase at his feet. He insisted that he didn't need any help leaving the hospital. However, after a chat about "rules being rules," he relented and let her wheel him to the elevator. On the way down, she asked him if his wife would be meeting him in the lobby. "I don't know," he said. "She's upstairs in the bathroom changing out of her hospital gown."

17

In the previous chapter, we talked about the stereotypes that exist today regarding old age; can you think of any? My list would include crippled, grumpy, and burdensome. Movies such as "Grumpy Old Men" reinforce that view. "Ugly" would be another negative assumption. When I apply the concept of physical unattractiveness to aging, I am reminded that I have a black, curly hair that happily grows amid the otherwise light brown hairs on my right eyebrow. It seems to evade my tweezers whenever I go after it. And how about the neck tissue that takes on a life of its own over time? One of my students said he was afraid to be seen in public around Thanksgiving! It's true that certain indignities can go hand-in-hand with aging, but my point is that there are plenty of teenagers and young adults beating themselves up over acne, cellulite, and other "imperfections" that should not dominate the mind or spirit. Healthy self-improvement is a worthy lifelong process.

IT'S TRUE THAT CERTAIN INDIGNITIES CAN GO
HAND-IN-HAND WITH AGING, BUT MY POINT IS
THAT THERE ARE PLENTY OF TEENAGERS AND
YOUNG ADULTS BEATING THEMSELVES UP OVER
ACNE, CELLULITE, AND OTHER "IMPERFECTIONS"
THAT SHOULD NOT DOMINATE THE MIND OR SPIRIT.

Forgetfulness is another negative characteristic that is perhaps applied too exclusively to the sixty-plus set. Frankly, my memory has had its good periods and bad ones throughout my entire lifetime. Years ago, I attended Dale Carnegie sessions to help me remember people's names. The trick was to associate a new person's name with something like his glasses, the print on his tie, or her hairstyle. My problem was that once the person changed clothes or whatever I had associated with the name, I was back where I'd started. Therefore, I do not accept that my memory has gotten any worse, although I still work at remembering people's names.

My husband and I often work as a team remembering facts. Just this morning, we were trying to recall lyrics from a song. Between the two of us, we did it. People of all ages must develop their own techniques because none of us is perfect. I have always liked lists and still do. The invention of the sticky pad is one to be celebrated. Even more significant perhaps is that now we can use our iPad or cell phone to remind us of dates, events, deadlines, etc.

I have to admit that for every trait listed that has been attributed to old people, there is a modicum of truth for some of us. Many people take these silly jokes and natural imperfections all too seriously. Yearning to stay "forever young," they turn to facelifts, tummy tucks, and breast enhancements to lift, suck in, or perk up various body parts. For every body part lifted, tucked, sucked in or perked up, there is another waiting for a "fix."

On the other hand, some of us "seniors" are frail and in poor health. Others, while healthy and relatively vibrant, have only invalid (read: in-valid, as in "not valid") references for old age. It's not all pretty and positive, but let's look at aging for what it is and what it can be–not for the debilitating emotional hang-up it has become for many Americans.

Wouldn't it be great if the fun loving eighty-five-year old were the norm? And what if wrinkles really DID feel like a mark of character, as opposed to a source of shame? Studies on avoiding the downsides of aging are relatively new. Let's now look at ways people around the world are dealing in a positive fashion with the aging process.

Avoiding the Downsides of Aging

There are a myriad of studies evolving on the "keys to longevity." One of them tracked 20,000 people who were adults age 45-79 in the UK. The findings were published in the Public Library of Science. A group of researchers led by Kay-Tee Khaw of Cambridge determined that people who adopted four practices would live an average of fourteen years longer than those who didn't. Those rules to live by are:

- Don't smoke.
- Eat lots of fruits and vegetables.
- Exercise regularly.
- Drink alcohol in moderation.

The first three habits are not new to healthy living, but moderate use of alcohol is relatively new to lists, particularly the use of red wine, for which I am especially grateful.

Older and perhaps more popular studies are: the Okinawa Centenarian Study; "Living to 100" and other publications by Thomas Perls; the works of George Vaillant from Harvard; and of course, those of Erik Erikson, all of which will be explored and applied in later chapters.

Key Characteristics of Centenarians

In 2008, Dan Buettner published his book *The Blue*

Zones, which presented his study of centenarians in Sardinia, Italy; Okinawa, Japan; Loma Linda, California; and the Nicoya Peninsula in Costa Rica. He developed what he calls "The Power Nine" or "common denominators" that are "patterned after the lifestyles of Blue Zone centenarians, but modified to fit the Western lifestyle."

Buettner's list encompasses diet and exercise, but in a gentler way than we "quick-fix" Americans generally desire and expect. For example, exercise for Buettner's centenarians is NOT lifting heavy weights at the gym an hour a day, five days a week. It IS moving normally throughout each day, whether that means working in the garden, walking on a beach, climbing stairs, doing yoga, caring for children, or whatever encompasses routine activity. Buettner's list highlights that eating in moderation is a high fiber event with little meat or processed foods. Drinking red wine made the list, yet, not surprisingly, in moderation.

Also on Buettner's centenarian common denominator list are traits relating to one's state of mind. For example, the "powerful" people are those who have a purpose, those who make a point of reducing stress, those who have faith in a higher power of sorts, and those who value family by developing meaningful long-term relationships throughout the generations. Buettner's ninth trait is having the "right tribe." That translates to being surrounded by those who share Blue Zone values. *The Blue Zones* is a wonderful read for those of you who are interested in the details of the research.

Another study of note is one completed by Dr. Pat Ward-Baker. This study identified the common characteristics of awesome people, age eighty-five and older. Hers was a qualitative longitudinal study, as opposed to a scientific statistical study. Dr. Ward-Baker delved into the lives of her eight remarkable subjects through repeated interviews with open-ended questions. She drew from research in biology, psychology, and the sociology of aging.

All of her subjects lived in the United States, and the study included both men and women. All were living ambitious and active lives. Among them were a farmer, a photographer, an actress, a philanthropist, a historian, a pioneer in the treatment of damaged voices, and business owners.

Dr. Ward-Baker's list of common characteristics appears below:

- **Lifestyle**—All were aware of the need for exercise. They walked and watched their food intake, but none did so obsessively. Some swam, golfed, danced, played tennis, or worked out. None smoked or abused alcohol. None were obese.

- **Resilience**—They shared an attitude that was adaptive, optimistic, persistent, and positive. All had suffered losses and setbacks, but they didn't let those things stop them over time.

- **Internal Guidance Forward**—They were internally grounded, with a feeling that outcomes would be successful. All were very independent. They had a freedom from the concern of whether people liked them and from the demands and frustrations of earlier roles in life.

- **Full Engagement in Life**—They did something that challenged them and brought forth their best while engaging new skills and competencies. They had something that gave purpose or meaning to life and looked at the broader picture beyond themselves. They were absorbed, not just "active."

- **Commitment to Lifelong Learning**–They were focused on learning with an attitude of *growing* older, not just getting older.

- **Sense of Humor**–All had a sense of humor and could indeed laugh at themselves and the situations around them.

Research is Research . . . All Good!

Both Buettner's and Ward-Baker's lists of common characteristics are credible because both are based on facts. Indeed, both seem based on common sense, but then, wouldn't we expect that of centenarians? There is no "eat only bacon" focus. In addition, both studies are headed by lifestyle-related imperatives. Sorry, there is no way around it: diet and exercise ARE important. We know that.

The studies have key differences as well. Buettner's work focused on a worldwide view of centenarians versus Ward-Baker's American study. Of course, the research process, subjects, and selection of subjects were different, yet both are comprehensive and scholarly in their own ways. It does strike me that Buettner's work stresses the concept of nurturing, as he discusses being engaged in families and communities. It has a "living in (and enjoying) the moment" message. Ward-Baker's research stresses independence and recognizes that pushing through losses is necessary over time. The latter values enjoying the moment, but not necessarily wallowing in it. Instead, Ward-Baker focuses on continual new learning and growth. Perhaps the differences are cultural; you can be the judge. As we concluded earlier, aging is an individual experience.

However you view the two research efforts, there is no data in either study that would suggest we spend the last twenty years of our lives in a chair—or worse, in bed in a rest home. Both studies confirm that we *can* live long, enjoyable, healthful lives, free of debilitating maladies. Remember that our goal is to keep rolling until just after our 120th birthday bash, when we suddenly die in our sleep or continue growing to 130.

Supercentenarian Wannabes

In the January 28, 2011 *Times-News* (Hendersonville, NC), there was an article about Boyd Campbell. Boyd was eighty when he started swimming competitively at the YMCA. He did so until he reached 100 and was subsequently sidelined by a broken hip. At 101, he was training to get back in the game! Local role models for our future exist if we seek them out—and accept them as being as normal as our "old" stereotypes.

It is time for those of us who have a vision of ourselves at age 100-plus as being independent, taking care of our health, staying engaged in life, continuing to plan and learn, and enjoying our family and friends, to have a presence as a group. We deserve a new focus on the growing numbers of folks who don't see themselves as "old and unable" and don't appreciate the labels that depict us in the negative. With our new vision in mind, we can now turn to our thoughts on how to get there.

3

LEADERSHIP DEVELOPMENT IN MIDLIFE

"WE TURN NOT OLDER WITH THE YEARS,
BUT NEWER EVERY DAY."
EMILY DICKINSON

What is Midlife?

Let us now begin to look at ourselves whatever age we are currently, and to consider how to get from here to our new vision of the centenarian we want to be. Often, even young adults are already beginning to look back and panic, thinking about what they have failed to accomplish, as opposed to the many possibilities the future holds. Changing our definition of "old" or "senior" requires a new view of midlife as well. People at all ages would do well to look forward to the future and to prepare for it with information and a positive attitude, not dread. Likewise, those approaching 100 can look forward, set goals, and continue to grow.

When I began my Ph.D. studies at age fifty-two, I started with a focus on organizational change, a subject near and dear to my heart, having led groups as large as 9,600 people. However, what I found was that with the freedom to study anything I wanted, I preferred to look ahead rather than to document what I'd done in corporate life.

With that "aha," I shifted my Ph.D. quest to an in-depth study of midlife leadership, supposing that one doesn't stop living or being at one's best just because one retires or turns some magical age that the government, in its wisdom, has deemed "Social Security eligible." It was also clear to me that my former role of business leader paled in comparison to the work I needed to do as a midlife aging leader/parent with three teenagers. I decided to perform an information-rich, qualitative analysis with eleven participants who exhibited exceptional midlife leadership qualities.

One doesn't stop living or being at one's best just because one retires or turns some magical age that the government, in its wisdom, has deemed "Social Security Eligible."

One of the dilemmas one faces when writing a Ph.D. dissertation is the meaning of words. I found over 850 definitions for "leadership" and no real consensus on "midlife." In the case of leadership, I felt at liberty to add yet another definition that would grow out of my studies. On the other hand, there were some significant scholars who had spent lifetimes defining and refining "midlife" development, although they may not have called it that. Erik Erikson was prominent among them. Erikson was a German psychologist whose greatest innovation was to postulate not five stages of development, as Sigmund Freud had done with his pyschosexual stages, but eight, adding three stages of adulthood. His widow, Joan Serson Erikson, elaborated on his model before her own death, adding a ninth stage (creatively, "old age") to it, taking into consideration the increasing life expectancy in Western cultures.

Each of Erikson's psychosocial stages is marked by a conflict (like trust versus mistrust) for which successful resolution will result in a favorable outcome. Erikson assigned favorable outcomes of each stage a "virtue." Erikson saw "middle adulthood" beginning at age forty and continuing to age sixty-five. He thought "maturity" would begin at sixty-five and last until death. The conflict we would wrestle with during "maturity" would be "integrity versus despair." The favorable outcome was "acceptance of one's life" and the virtue was "wisdom." His wife thought her stage of "old age" began at eighty-five. She saw the conflict as "apathy versus creativity" with a favorable outcome of "spiritual transcendence." There was no "virtue" assigned to this stage, which I found lacking.

Erikson's studies provide one source to think about when we look at our own development over time. To keep things simple, however, and once again recognizing that we are all living longer these days, for our purposes we could consider "midlife" anywhere from forty to ninety. Yet, once again, that is determined to a degree by each individual. When we assign a numerical range, we beg the question, "What happens after age ninety?" Is it fair or just to call someone like Boyd Campbell "old" when he is swimming competitively at age one hundred?

With that thought in mind, let's look at "midlife" *without* specific numerical boundaries. Susan Wittig Albert, author of *Writing from Life*, describes midlife as "turning from the outer to the inner self." Through much research, numerous interviews, and courses conducted throughout the United States and Mexico, as well as an incredible internship that led to my next career working with clients on midlife transitions, I constructed a process for leadership development in midlife. It proposes that "midlife" is when we do indeed turn from the outer to the inner self, as Albert has suggested. Absolute age becomes superfluous in my model.

Leadership Development in Midlife

The process for Leadership in Midlife that we will discuss involves four steps:

1. Positioning for Change (moving from a "quick fix" to the journey)
2. Self Discovery (finding balance in a life of compulsive behaviors)
3. A Broader Sense of Purpose (living through principles)
4. Pursuit of Unique Potential (the self in connection)

The process is staged with a natural flow. We will start by positioning ourselves for the inner journey ahead, along with the inevitable challenges it will bring. In Step Two, we explore our ideals and even imperfections that make us the incredible beings we are. In Step Three, you will form a new broad sense of purpose that works for you. The process then evolves to Step Four where we introspectively map out connections to our unique potential.

I first heard the term "unique potential" in a family program at the Hyde School, a remarkable prep school our oldest son attended for three years, along with our daughter who attended for a shorter period. The school distinguished itself by two main things: one was that it was "character" based and as such, its leaders developed all activities around five values—courage, integrity, leadership, curiosity, and concern; the second was its requirement that parents go to school in Hyde's "family program" at the same time their children are at the school. Joe Gauld, the founder of Hyde, believes that the main job of parents is to inspire their children. He also believes that parents should be "spiritual parents." In other words, a spiritual parent would "accept that his or her child has a purpose and a destiny dictated by a higher power." The same is true for all of us whether we have had children or not. We were all children ourselves at one time, even if we find that hard to recall now.

Others describe "character" a bit more expansively than Hyde, making it sound more like how I would define "unique potential." William James once said, "I have often thought that the best way to define a man's character would be to seek out the particular mental or moral attitude in which, when it came upon him, he felt himself most deeply and intensively active and alive. At such moments, there is a voice inside that speaks and says, 'This is the real me.'"

And so it is with your unique potential . . . it is the real you. It is what Leider in 1996 called "self leadership: the ultimate leadership task." Warren Bennis says it another way: "Becoming a leader is synonymous with becoming yourself."

4

STEP ONE:
POSITIONING FOR CHANGE
Moving from the "Quick Fix" to the Journey

"YOU MUST DO THE THING
YOU THINK YOU CANNOT DO."
ELEANOR ROOSEVELT

I struggle to bring myself from a world of instant grati-
fication and "quick fixes" to one focused on the journey
through life. My "quick fixes" have included crazy diet
plans, which never worked long term, and vacations de-
signed to "get away from it all." I always found that "all of
it" was still there–and sometimes more troublesome–when
I returned from vacation and that in general, short-term
thinking to satisfy a problem of the moment without regard for the long-term consequence never solves anything.

I even tried to apply a "quick fix" mentality to raising
my children. Our first son, God bless him, was born when
the "Super Mom" concept was taking shape. We were
women who had not only a husband and children, but
also high-powered careers outside the home. Some of us
may remember the "Enjoli woman" in the 1980 commer-
cial advertising a perfume by Charles of Ritz "for the 24-
hour woman." We could do anything quickly, we thought,
and make it look easy.

When my son was eighteen months old, I took Dr.

Spock's advice that that was the perfect age to potty train him. However, my method was quite different from the ones he recommended. I found a book called *Toilet Training in a Weekend* that would act as my guide. I bought the necessary gear, which included a miniature plastic potty, a rubber doll that would pee when "fed," the doll's water bottle, and my son's favorite juice. I then settled into the kitchen with my adorable, innocent little son.

The idea was that my son would feed the baby doll and then put him on the potty where the doll would "relieve" itself. In turn, I would feed my son lots of juice, and when he needed to go, we would race down to the "big boys' potty," and my son would go.

Can you believe I did this? The irony is that it actually worked. Whatever I did in the process that shaped my son's view of life would be something I don't even want to think about. Fortunately, the experience has not prevented him from turning into a terrific young adult–in spite of me!

I have fond memories of sitting on the floor beside my second son when he was in the learning mode on the potty, reading Richard Scarry's *"Cars and Trucks and Things That Go"* to find the mischievous Goldbug, a completely opposite approach from a "quick fix." It may have taken longer, but it concluded with far less guilt on my part. Our third child, our daughter, somehow just figured it all out without an elaborate process of any kind that I recall. I'm sure the fact that I was less anxious played a role in her growth.

My own struggle with "quick fixes" crops up here and there to this day. Two years ago, I incurred a torn meniscus in my knee while playing tennis. I opted for surgery right away, even though in retrospect, some doctors now recommend that people who are not in pain might want to wait to see if the tear heals on its own. Thus, I ask myself, *Have I once and for all learned my lesson?* We'll see, but I think I'm making progress, one mistake at a time. As someone once said, "What's the sense in making mistakes if we don't learn from them?" We all are works in progress.

Understand then, that even though we are taking you adventurous souls through the "leadership development in midlife" process in 120 pages, in the wonderful world of "quick fixes" we've all grown up in–THIS IS NO QUICK FIX! There is no pill to take, no surgery available, no easy way to jump to the end. This is a beginning for the here and now.

And so, here we are positioning for change. As we begin, let's consider the "120-Year Plan" in a nutshell. We can draw a line on a piece of paper that represents our 120-year lifespan. There will be the word "born" at the beginning of the line, and our goal "120" at the end. We now begin to change a paradigm about how long we might live. Goals matter! For example, recently, I learned that a friend of ours had passed away at age eighty-seven. For as long as we knew him, his stated goal was to outlive his father, who had died at eighty-six. He literally "let go" after that: he met his goal. Another recent example in the *Greenville News* talked about Lillie Watson, who at 101 years of age, wanted to make her "exit" after the new year. She passed away on the first day of January at 1:20 a.m. As Henry Ford once said, "Whether you think you can or think you can't, you're right."

On a personal level, if I think I'm going to live to seventy, I'm going to spend my time, not to mention my money, in a very different way than if I think I'm good for 120. Think about this for a moment: What would you do if you knew with certainty that you would live only one more year? What about ten years? Or forty years? What would be your considerations?

Let's raise the ante here. By virtue of reading this book,

you are officially on the 120-year plan. Your line is drawn and will represent your timeline. When you were born, you brought with you a host of genes, traits, preferences, skills, talents, likes, and dislikes which were inherited from your parents and ancestors, many of whom you may never have met. This amalgamation that becomes you at birth represents a unique combination never seen before in a newborn.

What we do with all that is then determined by our attitude, family values, education, interactions with others, health circumstances, jobs we hold, and so on. You can plot some of these life events on your timeline such as birth, the start and end of formal education, your first job, retirement if relevant, etc. During all those years, there were expectations for our busy lives. Fill in events until your line brings you into the present.

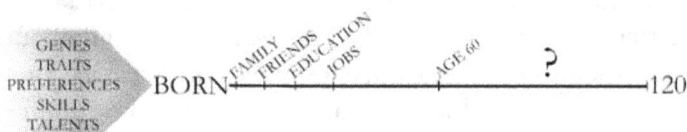

THE 120-YEAR PLAN

I happen to be sixty-six, and I am at that point on my timeline with fifty-four more years left before I reach 120. I was fifty-two the first time I drew that line with more years left to live than I had already experienced. It seemed to me that expectations were clear for the first half of my life, but solidly muddy for the second half. I know it's the same way for many others. With that said, the objective for the 120-year plan is to have a fulfilling 120 years with as little sickness as possible before we "pass on" in our sleep after our 120th year birthday. Someone once said, "Good health is merely the slowest possible rate at which one can die." That's our goal; so how do we do that and what fills

34

in those remaining years which potentially could be as many as we've already lived—or more?

SOMEONE ONCE SAID,
"GOOD HEALTH IS MERELY THE SLOWEST POSSIBLE RATE AT WHICH ONE CAN DIE."

Slow Growth or Deep Change?

Belgian physicist Ilya Prigogine was awarded a Nobel Prize for his theory of "dissipative structures," part of which contends that friction is a fundamental property of nature and nothing grows without it. Let's begin with some thoughts on change and growth. What are some words that come to mind when you consider change? Others before you have suggested such things as "alter, modify, vary, transform, revolutionize, adjust, amend, hard, difficult, don't like, adaptation, crisis, and transition." Webster's Dictionary defines change as "the act, process, or result of changing" . . . now THAT'S really helpful. Reading on, we come to "transformation," "alteration," and "substitution."

And how about growth? Others before you have suggested such synonyms as "enlargement, expansion, development, augmentation, intensification, escalation, learning, and new ideas." Webster once again is helpful as he says that growth is a "stage in the process of growing." The definition continues with "progressive development," "evolution," "increase," and "expansion."

The question is: can we have growth without change? I think not. Robert Quinn, in one of my favorite books, *Deep Change*, says that we only have two choices in life—deep change or slow death. Every day when we get up we can ask ourselves, "Is this a day of slow death or deep change?"

ROBERT QUINN, IN ONE OF MY FAVORITE BOOKS, *DEEP CHANGE*, SAYS THAT WE ONLY HAVE TWO CHOICES IN LIFE—DEEP CHANGE OR SLOW DEATH.

Looking at this another way, while traveling in Australia, we stayed at a charming little bed and breakfast in Cairns. The grounds of the property were lovely with a variety of flowers and plants throughout, obviously cared for with love. While we were talking with the owner about her experiences and transitions in life, she said, "We all need repotting over time!"

Both deep change and repotting spawn new growth, yet both require risk. What if our change or repotting doesn't work?

The Ultimate Risk

My husband and I spend our summers in Maine, a state known for lobsters. Think about the fact that in order for a lobster to grow, it has to shed that shell that protects it from predators. Lobsters literally have to subject themselves to the ultimate risk, the threat of death, to grow. Sometimes when I take risks, it can feel like that to me as well.

Taking risks was made vivid to me while my son was at the Hyde School and parents and children were challenged to cross over a rather swampy body of water called the "duck pond" by hanging from a rope strung between two trees on either side of the pond. The first summer at a parent-child retreat, I was the only parent that didn't attempt the exercise. At the time, I felt that I didn't need to prove myself to anyone by hanging from a rope. Truth be known, I was scared to death to take a risk that was totally out of my comfort zone. Needless to say, my son was devastated.

Through much self-examination following the incident, I realized that I had basically stopped taking risks in my life. The "duck pond" experience became a symbol for me. I had become extremely complacent in life, not caring to—or wanting to—change things, thus holding myself back from sorely needed growth. Although I was working very hard at my job, my family life was falling apart around me.

As a result of that experience, I realized that in order to change my workaholic ways, which were rewarded in my work environment and too long a part of who I was, I would need to take a risk and retire from my company after twenty-seven years. I could not see myself saving my family if I didn't change my environment. My work had taken the place of my family as my number one priority. I had to leave my job and my lucrative salary behind to place family where they should be.

Thinking about this now, I see that I had realized that my own plans and will weren't working out so well, and "if I continued to do what I'd always done, I'd get what I had always gotten," as some might say. Frankly, that wasn't working for me—or my family. My family deserved to be number one.

I did make the transition to a new company, promising myself that I would no longer travel long distances from home, no longer bring work home every night and weekend, and that I would arrive at work at eight o'clock in the morning and leave by six in the evening. I essentially kept that promise.

The following year, our family went back to the summer session at Hyde. This time, I vowed to cross the duck pond. Although I waited until the last possible minute to put on my helmet and climb the tree to the rope that hung across the pond, I made myself get out there and move across the rope. In truth, I probably would have avoided the whole thing again—had I not been challenged by another parent who said he would watch me do it. Anyway, with seemingly no choice left, off we went, my husband, daughter, and one son in tow.

About three quarters of the way across the pond, my arms and legs let go, and I fell into the muck. As I struggled to come out of the water, I heard my son yell out, "You did good, Mom!" Nirvana. My daughter also was excited. Maybe I hadn't gotten all the way across, but I took the risk. Shortly thereafter, my son turned a corner and became a leader on campus, having great success on the athletic field, in academics, and in his college search. He had finally seen, as did my daughter, that even Mom was not perfect and had her own struggles to confront. Our family was on the mend at last.

I'm guessing that, like me, you also see taking risks and changing ways as hard. We can illustrate that point with a little exercise. Simply fold your arms in front of you as you normally would. Note which hand is up and which hand is down. Now flip them so that the hand that's up is down and the hand that's down is up. How does that feel? Most people would say that it feels uncomfortable, tough, or even weird. Some have difficulty doing it at all. Change is hard, often seen as risky and not something we commonly reach out for in life.

Why is change something we avoid or maybe even fear in our lives? Do you have a fear that holds you back? I have a fear of heights. Some years ago, when the children were still young, my husband decided to take up hot air ballooning (of all things), flying out of our back yard with friends.

Eventually, he earned a pilot's license and bought a hot air balloon company shortly after my experience at the duck pond. Do you think that I could then avoid going up in that tiny basket to see what the thrill was all about? Believe me, I tried. However, it was clear that I needed to face my fear and get up there. I must say, it was quite the experience. I loved floating over the treetops and watching people rush out of their homes with their morning coffee to see what was going on above them. It was indeed a beautiful sight all around. Today, I am grateful for the experience and personal growth that came with that trip.

Linking Change and Growth

Let's look at the question, "Can we have growth without change?" another way.

Get a piece of paper and grab a pencil. Take a minute to list some of what you'd call "major changes" in your life and the characteristics associated with those changes; that is, why you changed and what was going on that caused a change. Divide a portion of the paper into three columns.

LINKING
CHANGE & GROWTH

MAJOR CHANGE	CAUSE	OUTCOME	GROWTH SPURT	CAUSE	OUTCOME

One column is entitled "Major Change," and beside it, in the next column is "Cause." A final column is entitled "Outcome." Think of three or more major changes in your life.

Now think about growth spurts in your life and the characteristics associated with those. When have you achieved greatest growth? Again, use three columns on your paper with headings "Growth Spurt," "Cause," and "Outcome." List three or more growth spurts you've experienced in your life along with their causes and outcomes.

When I have done this exercise in groups, often the major changes coincide with the growth spurts. For example, one participant noted his move to Africa. The cause was an "urge." His outcome was an appreciation for a dramatically different cultural environment. Many participants also will list getting an education as both change and growth. Marriage, divorce, having children, and changing careers can appear as either major changes or growth spurts—commonly both—in one's life. One of my participants made the observation that if you are taking a risk, what you are really saying is, "I believe in tomorrow, and I will be a part of it."

For years, on my bedroom mirror, I had a yellow Post-it note on which I had written, "When you struggle, you grow!" I wanted to grow, but I hated the struggle. Indeed, some things never change.

Let us now turn to our self-discovery step with the thought that our midlife leadership development process is not intended to be a "quick fix," but rather intended to facilitate our journey in life. Hopefully you have chosen to pursue deep change and growth over the alternatives and are now ready to look at yourself in an introspective fashion.

5

STEP TWO: SELF DISCOVERY
Finding Balance in a Life of
Compulsive Behaviors

"THE LONGEST JOURNEY IS THE JOURNEY INWARD."
DAG HAMMARSKJOLD

Each of us was introduced to the important concept of balance at birth . . . two arms, two eyes, two legs, etc. That concept may have been reinforced by things like the "Hokey Pokey" in elementary school gym class. Over time, we have undoubtedly appreciated the fact that we have two arms and two legs. Having had both a broken right wrist and a broken left ankle, I can speak first hand to the value of having a second limb to rely on during the healing process.

Yoga instructors I work with certainly understand the importance of balance and keep us on our toes about the subject. Yet, for some reason, I was still surprised when I went to physical therapy after surgery for the torn meniscus in my right knee; the therapist had me do everything I was doing on the right leg with my left leg as well in order to maintain balance.

The principle of Feng Shui is based on the ancient Taoist concept of energetic polarity. It is the study of energy meridians that crisscross the earth and the practice of aligning them. The terms "yin and yang" describe the opposite yet complementary energy states in the universe.

Yin is the negative pole of North and West (sunset), and yang is the positive pole South and East (sunrise). Yin activities might be sleeping, taking a hot bath, getting a foot message, reading, or meditating. Yang activities would be exercising, cooking, studying, or being actively engaged in a hobby. For those of you building or remodeling homes, Feng Shui would also go on to suggest that bedrooms and bathrooms might best be placed in the northern or western parts of the house, and office, kitchen, living room, and dining room, in the southern and eastern parts of the house. And we thought it was all about the view!

The Yellow Emperor who was the first ruler of China some 4,700 years ago was said to have pondered the concept of balance versus indulgence as it related to longevity. In *The Yellow Emperor's Classic of Medicine*, we see the observation that people who "ate balanced diets at regular times, arose and retired at regular hours, avoided overburdening minds and bodies, and refrained from overindulgences of all kinds . . . maintained well-being in mind and body and often lived past 100 years." Of course, we have no way of knowing how accurate his records were, yet his point is a valid one.

We learn from Dr. Maoshing Ni's book *Secrets of Longevity*, that in Eastern studies, it is believed that a balance between the polarities can help one stay in energy alignment and lead a healthy life. On the other hand, Dr. Ni goes on to say that "People have changed their ways. They drink wine like water, indulge in excessive eating . . . drain their essence and deplete their energy. Seeking emotional excitement and momentary pleasures, people disregard the natural rhythm and order of the universe. They fail to regulate their lifestyle and diet, and they sleep improperly. They do not know the secrets of conserving their energy and vitality. So it is not surprising that they look old at fifty . . . "

The Spiral of Change
Learning from Nature

Nature teaches us a lot about change and balance. Think about the four seasons of the year. The fall and winter are yin periods, while summer and spring are yang periods. The changing of the seasons is also a conditioning for the change we talked about earlier.

Think of it like this: We peak in our careers when our income is at a high, or in our family life when our children are "on their own." We're in the summer of our lives. All our hard work is paying off.

Then we move into the fall season with a slip-sliding effect. We might feel lost or feel like we've lost our identity. Perhaps we have retired or are now "empty nested" and have a lot of time on our hands. We slide into winter where we cocoon and perhaps fall into depression, particularly if we stay there too long. Menopause can often do that to women; midlife crisis for men. By contrast, in nature, trees need that time of winter to conserve energy and get ready for what follows. That is what winter or that cocooning period is meant to be–a restorative, contemplative period–in human terms.

Then comes a rebirth in spring when buds come out and for us, in this analogy, new ideas are put into action. Perhaps we move to a new community, go back to school, change careers, volunteer doing something we like, or follow a passion.

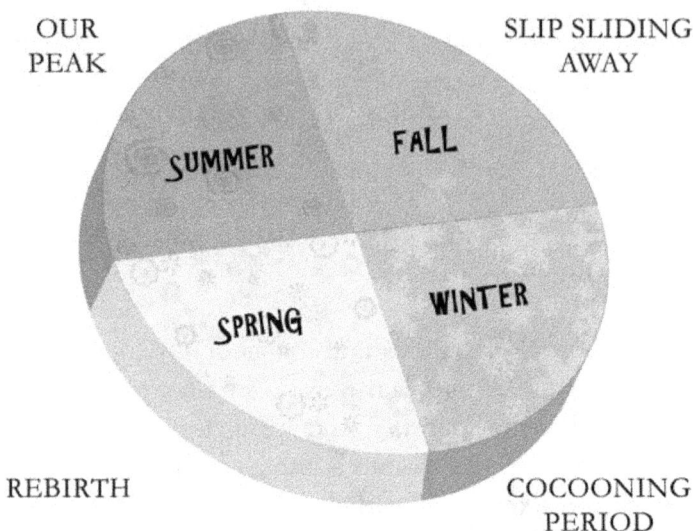

OUR PEAK

SLIP SLIDING AWAY

SUMMER

FALL

SPRING

WINTER

REBIRTH

COCOONING PERIOD

THE SEASONS OF OUR LIVES

An example of my own "winter" identity crisis came after I had left my second major role in corporate America to "retire." Although I had had some rather lofty titles and many acquaintances in corporate life, I was now relegated to doing normal everyday functions such as grocery shopping. I was in line at a grocery store and suddenly realized that I knew no one and certainly had no power to go to the front of the line. What a strange feeling that was. My sense of identity had disappeared. When I finally made it back to my car, I cried for quite some time. That was the day I made my first personal set of business cards, entitling myself "President and CEO" to establish a new identity. I felt I needed to BE someone or something. I became a consultant in a field very familiar to me. The good part of that was that it was a healthy income for a period of six months. However, I abhorred the work and knew I needed to move on.

Around that six-month mark, I had the good fortune of facilitating a seminar with parents and their teenagers. One father was upset and telling the group that he was losing his business, and he kept asking, "Who will I be if I'm not the CEO of this firm?" His son, also upset, said, "You'll be my dad. You'll always be my dad."

I couldn't get that scene out of my mind. I kept asking myself, "Who am I REALLY, once I strip off all the roles I play?" Once I arrived home, I made a new set of business cards. My new title was "A Real Person." That one felt right. Mark Sanborn, author of *You Don't Need a Title to Be a Leader,* would appreciate that story.

Take Hold and Let Go

On a smaller scale, we go through this spiral of change through our own seasons repeatedly over time. Think of it as a corkscrew of sorts as we turn and twist it further within.

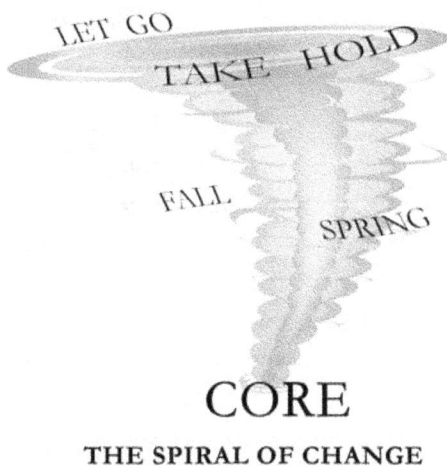

LET GO

TAKE HOLD

FALL

SPRING

CORE

THE SPIRAL OF CHANGE

We let go of something (call it fall) and take hold of something else (call it spring) with each turn. If we try to take hold of the new before we let go of the old, we find ourselves pulled and in emotional straits. Have you ever balanced on high ropes strung between trees? One of those exercises I observed had ropes hanging vertically above at six-foot intervals. In order to take hold of the next rope, a participant literally had to let go of the one he or she had in hand while continuing to balance on the rope underfoot. That concept was true for me when I ultimately left my work in corporate life and went back to school for my Ph.D. In order to grow once again, I needed to let go of my existing situation.

IF WE TRY TO TAKE HOLD OF THE NEW BEFORE WE LET GO OF THE OLD, WE FIND OURSELVES PULLED AND IN EMOTIONAL STRAITS.

Moving Closer to Your Core

Over time, the ideal spiral brings us closer to our core, what's really important in our lives, which we will explore. It is critical to keep in mind that perfection is not our goal. We're looking for progress, not perfection. I am reminded that the great ancient Chinese artists always included a deliberate flaw in their work to emphasize that human creation is never perfect. Our journey is a process, and we still need to grow. Remember, no "quick fixes." We're searching for what we're supposed to be doing with our lives. Stay tuned until we get to our chapter on sense of purpose.

Obsessions and Addictions

Now let's look at the opposite of balance, another yin and yang mentioned earlier by Dr. Ni. We can call it an obsession or addiction such as overindulgent eating, workaholism, need for perfection, desire to "have it all," etc. When I look back at my life, I find I've had a lot of obsessions. As a young child, I was addicted to donuts, hot out of the oil from the local A&P grocery store, and I would brag about eating as many as seven of them for breakfast. No wonder they called me "Fatty Patty"! On a larger scale, I would eat lots of everything, especially dessert. My mom was a fantastic cook.

As a teenager, I went the other way and starved myself, subscribing to every new fad diet that came out. I was obsessed with thinness, so much so that my body no longer allowed me to menstruate. I took my addictive behavior into corporate life, where I was a workaholic extraordinaire, often sleeping no more than two hours a night. I was addicted to perfection—having it all, doing it all, and doing it perfectly. I knew I couldn't snap my fingers and make it rain, but I did feel a certain God-like control over everyday circumstances. The truth was that I was merely working harder to quell the anxiety of my addictions while perpetuating them.

For the first time in my life, I now finally feel in a better state of balance. A couple of years ago, I managed to wean myself off of an addiction to M&M's, but I need to recognize that I have an addictive personality and can easily slip again. What sometimes rings in my ears is a comment made by a participant in my class three years ago. The very active gentleman was ninety-three years old. He said, "People ask me what my secret is . . . it's moderation."

Take a minute now to think about your own addictions over time and write them down on a piece of paper. What have you come up with? How do you think addictions make you feel?

Life Balance Exercise

Now let's do a little exercise to see how balanced we are (or aren't) in life.

The International Council on Active Aging (ICAA) invented the phrase "Active Aging" to describe the process of one who is engaged in life. The term is used to depict people who live life as fully as possible within six dimensions of wellness:

- Intellectual (mind growth)
- Physical (working on your physical self)
- Social (time with family and friends)
- Emotional (inner healing and study)
- Spiritual (time spent thinking about who you are and who you're becoming)
- Vocational (could be employment or volunteering for a cause or interest)

We look at each dimension to simplify our understanding during this exercise, but we understand that the dimensions do, in fact, intertwine in our lives and do not act as separate components. Actually, there have been times in my life during which I felt I had only four components: sleeping, working, eating, and looking for things I had just seen a minute ago. However, we will go with the aforementioned six.

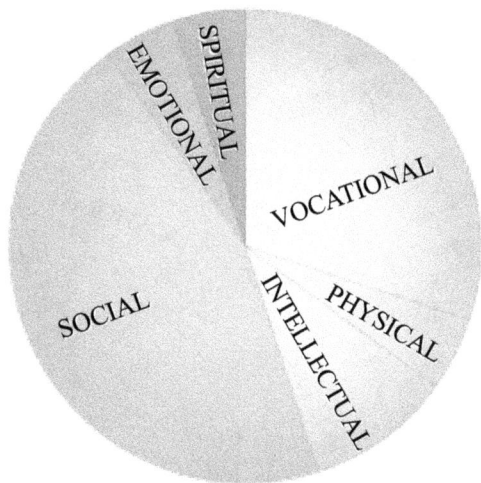

EXAMPLE OF LIFE TODAY

Draw a circle on a piece of paper. Thinking about your life today, divide your circle or pie into six pieces (Intellectual, Physical, Social, Emotional, Spiritual, and Vocational) with a small slice representing a small part of your time dedicated to that component, and a larger piece used to indicate a larger amount of your time. Try to make them somewhat representative of your overall life this past year, so I would not be surprised if I looked at your pie and compared it to your calendar of activities.

Now draw another circle, and this time, divide the pie pieces the way you would like your life to be.

Think about what you came up with. Where are the areas you spend most of your time? Which are those you neglect? To achieve balance, what changes would be required? Our next several chapters will deal with each of those six components in life in more detail to help you in answering those questions.

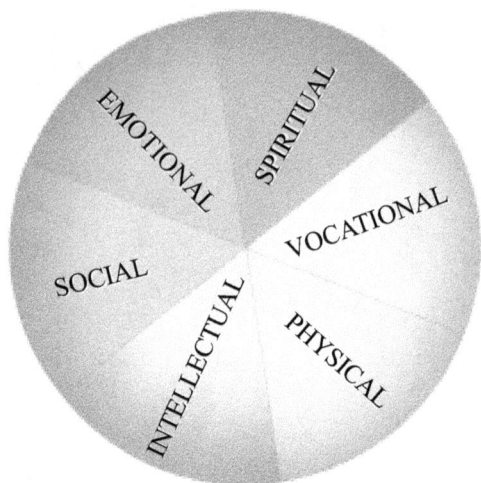

A LIFE IN BALANCE

Another extremely helpful self-analysis, which I highly recommend you do if you haven't already, or haven't done lately, is either a Myers-Briggs test or the Keirsey Temperament Test. They can be found online using your favorite search engine. Both identify sixteen personality preferences, one of which will fit you. Having done both tests in the past year, I can tell you that the results were the same. I find the Keirsey test is less expensive (it used to be free), takes less time (about fifteen minutes to complete) and is a good representation of your current personality state. When you select your answers, pick the first thing that strikes you. Don't over-think the questions, and try not to change any answers. There is no right or wrong. This will be an important step in your discovery of self as you are today.

Often companies will ask employees to take these tests to help in selecting the right people for positions or to assist with teamwork interplay. When I first took the Myers-Briggs test in my thirties, I was an "ESTJ." I was extroverted, rule-bound, careful of duties and responsibilities, and results oriented. I liked facts, with a thought process oriented around logic.

What I have learned is that over time, often our preferences, particularly as they relate to the middle two letters, S (Sensing) versus N (Intuition), and T (Thinking) versus F (Feeling), can change. This often happens in midlife contributing to, or perhaps causing, our midlife "crisis."

Sometime in my early fifties, I became an "ENFJ." I am still extroverted, which means I get my energy from being around people, as opposed to being by myself. However, I now easily imagine the possibilities in reaching goals without compromising my personal code of ethics. My conscience guides me, rather than a list of rules. My feelings, which were set aside in the business environment as a form of survival as a woman at the time, are now the driver of my behavior, as opposed to pure logic and facts. That is not to say that I don't still use facts and logic in my thought process; they are simply no longer the dominant choice.

Self-discovery, of course, is just that–discovering who we really are over time. We each do it in our own way. I strongly recommend that you take advantage of the tools available to help you with that process. I have found that it is also interesting for the entire family to take the same tests, collectively discuss results, and chat about what that might mean to family interaction. Doing so will surely ignite lively conversations at the dinner table.

Blowing Through Genetics

Before we get into the material dealing with the six afore-mentioned component areas of our lives, we should address the rather widely held concept that our longevity is destined by our ancestors. That is, if our parents lived into their nineties, we will as well. Likewise, many feel that if their parents passed away early in life, they are doomed. Research refutes those arguments. It has determined that genetics contribute only 25-30 percent to the causative factors behind length and quality of life. A famous study assessing Danish twins in two different environments has proven that point with an examination of nature versus nurture. Other studies have authenticated those results. It's nice if you have a long history of people in your family living until well over 100, and that certainly doesn't hurt, but it is NOT the determining factor we used to assume it was. What really counts is what we do with what we have: the balance of our intellectual stimulation, physical well-being, social networking, emotional literacy, spiritual growth, and vocational desires. We will look at each area in more detail.

WHAT REALLY COUNTS IS WHAT WE DO WITH WHAT WE HAVE: THE BALANCE OF OUR INTELLECTUAL STIMULATION, PHYSICAL WELL BEING, SOCIAL NETWORKING, EMOTIONAL LITERACY, SPIRITUAL GROWTH, AND VOCATIONAL DESIRES.

6

INTELLECTUAL STIMULATION

"WE ARE THE SUM TOTAL OF OUR THOUGHTS."
RALPH WALDO EMERSON

Go back to the growth spurts in your life. Did any of them occur in some form of school or new learning environment? What new learning are you involved in today? Do you want to enhance the time you spend on intellectual growth? And what is intellectual growth, anyway? How do we get it?

I had thought when I went back for my Ph.D. at fifty-two years of age that I would be the oldest one in the group. Little did I know that our instructor would be in her eighties and that several of my classmates were in their late sixties or seventies, which, admittedly, I thought was "old" at the time; now that I am almost there, I don't feel a day over thirty-five! I embarked on the additional schooling effort because, at the time, I was craving new growth. I equated going back to school with intellectual stimulation. It turned out to be only the beginning . . .

The Power of Thought

There was an article in *The Wall Street Journal* on January 19, 2007, that discussed how thinking can change the brain. The writer described what the Dalai Lama is doing to help scientists see the power of the mind in shaping grey matter. Apparently for years, neuroscientists had explained to him that mental experiences reflect chemical and electrical changes in the brain. When electrical impulses zip through our visual cortex, for example, we see. The Dalai Lama wondered if, in addition to the brain giving rise to thoughts, hopes, beliefs, and emotions that add up to this thing we call the brain, might not the brain cause physical changes in the very matter that created it? If so, pure thought would change the brain's activities, its circuits or even its structures. Could specific, subtle thoughts influence the brain?

In studies done by scientists since, looking at the brains of monks trained in meditation, they found evidence that mental training can indeed create an enduring brain trait. The findings, according to a Dr. Richard J. Davidson at the University of Wisconsin, "clearly indicate that meditation can change the function of the brain in an enduring way." Furthermore, findings in additional studies demonstrate that a short program in mindfulness meditation produces demonstrable effects on brain and immunity functions. These findings suggest that meditation may change brain and immunity functions in positive ways and underscore the need for additional research."

"In our country people are very involved in the physical-fitness craze, working out several times a week," says Davidson. "But we don't pay that kind of attention to our minds. Modern neuroscience is showing that our minds are as plastic as our bodies. Meditation can help you train your mind, in the same way exercise can train your body."

Davidson's research didn't stop with the monks. To find out whether meditation could have lasting, beneficial effects in the workplace, he performed a study at Madison Biotech Company. Four dozen employees met once a week for eight weeks to practice mindfulness. Davidson wrote, "The employees' left pre-fontal cortices were enlarged, just like those of the monks (but not as much by comparison)." And thus Davidson concluded that meditation can actually sculpt the brain.

The Mind and Visions

The mind is where our visions begin. Recently, I spoke with a friend, who has had a lingering health issue. She has been tested repeatedly and has been on medication for the condition for some time. Several months back, she decided to start meditating each day for 10-15 minutes to clear her mind of racing thoughts. At her last appointment with the doctor, who had been weaning her off the medication, he asked her what she had done because her tests were now normal. She said that the only change in her life has been her daily meditation. That's a "wow" for me.

Laugh Lines

Frankly, what I love best about meditation is that it makes doing nothing seem quite respectable.

Beyond meditation, certainly education and learning fight brain/mind compression by creating more connections in the brain. Anything you do to stimulate the mind can help. Reading, doing crossword puzzles, playing bridge, traveling, using a new technology, etc.–all of it counts. Recently, studies have shown that exercise also stimulates the brain. Personally, I love it when I can do one thing and get the benefit of two. I'm sure you can come up with your own list of ways to get your brain clicking. Keep in mind that one of the key characteristics of outstanding centenarians is "lifelong learning."

7

PHYSICAL WELL BEING

"WHEN YOU LEAN OVER TO PICK SOMETHING UP,
SEE IF THERE IS ANYTHING ELSE YOU CAN DO WHILE
YOU'RE DOWN THERE."
CHARLOTTE RUBENS BLOOMBERG

Minuses and Plusses

What do you think is our number one PREVENTABLE physical killer? Smoking is the answer. Recently, I lost both a very good friend and a cousin to lung cancer. Both had been heavy smokers. We all must know by now that smoking often kills people. If you haven't already started, don't. If you do smoke, stop.

Beyond that, there is a ton of literature out there describing what we all should be doing to address physical well being.

Most literature recommends smaller nutritional meals, less red meat, a diet high in unsaturated fats and low in trans fats, reduced salt intake, and more fish (especially the kind with high Omega 3, such as wild salmon). It is also widely accepted that we need to get seven to eight hours of sleep a night and exercise.

Drinking a glass of red wine a day is a relatively new recommendation and my personal favorite. As more research is done on red wine, however, particularly as it relates to centenarians in Sardinia and southwest France, it becomes clear that the red wine we drink isn't just ANY red wine. I knew there was a catch! Roger Corder, author of *The Red Wine Diet*, has spent years researching the "health-giving" benefits of wine. He found that wine drinkers have a lower incidence of heart disease and diabetes and are also less likely to suffer from dementia in old age.

Laugh Lines

One Sunday, a Southern minister decided that a visual demonstration would add emphasis to his sermon. With that in mind, he placed four worms into four separate jars.

The first worm was put into a container of alcohol. The second worm was put into a container of cigarette smoke. The third worm was put into a container of chocolate syrup. The fourth worm was put into a container of good clean soil.

At the conclusion of the sermon, the minister reported the following results:

The first worm in alcohol was dead.

The second worm in smoke was dead.

The third worm in chocolate syrup was dead.

The fourth worm in good clean soil was alive.

So the minister asked the congregation,"What can you learn from this demonstration?" Ethel, in the back of the room, raised her hand and said, "As long as you drink, smoke, and eat chocolate, you won't have worms." That pretty much ended the service.

According to Corder, wines from areas where people are living longer contain significantly higher levels of procyanidins found in grape skins and seeds.

In Corder's studies, "the grape yielding the most procyanidin-rich wines is Tannat, one of the grapes found in southwest France." However, other tests he has performed have found certain cabernets, malbecs, sangiovese, chiantis, and other grape varieties also have high concentrations, depending on where and how the grapes are grown, and the fermentation process used when making the wine. Apparently, low-yielding older vines in high altitudes produce the favored grapes. A long fermentation process is also required. To make this all a bit less tedious, he recommends we look for a label that speaks to "concentrated fruit flavors, with great acidity and a fine, full tannic finish with good aging potential." For those looking for a non-alcoholic alternative, try broccoli, cranberries, walnuts, blueberries, apples, and other "superfoods."

I like the above recommendations because they are common sense. They also track with the habits of our centenarians. However, there are many other studies that are not as strongly corroborated, yet hope to claim fame. One I bet you haven't heard about is chewing a pine bark extract called Pyenogenol. A study done at the University of Arizona with Type 2 Diabetes patients found that 60 percent of the participants ingesting the extract after twelve weeks were able to cut their blood pressure medication in half. Apparently, it has also reduced osteoarthritis joint pain and stiffness as well. In addition, I recently heard that coconut oil has been shown to help in prevention of Alzheimer's disease. I like coconut oil (yet am less likely to chew pine bark even though it is handy where I live), but I think I'll wait for more studies before I jump on those bandwagons. Tested, tried, and true over time works for me.

Feeling Full on Fiber

The best book I have found on improving physical health is *The Gene Smart Diet* by Dr. Floyd Chilton. Again, no fads, just common sense backed up by a lot of research. If you want to lose weight, feel better, enhance your immune system, and always feel "full," this is your guide.

My husband and I are physically active but had reached a plateau on weight when we first read the book. No matter what we did, our weight stayed the same or went up, and we were always hungry. I hadn't been eating a regular lunch in years. Two years ago, when we started focusing on eating high fiber, "gene smart" foods, Warren lost ten pounds and I lost seven–and the best part is that we weren't even trying. At that point, weight loss was not the goal; improving metabolism and feeling full were the goals. Amazing to me was that by having a healthy lunch, with fruit and/or vegetables, and switching from red meat to fish rich in Omega 3, I lost weight and improved my resting metabolism rate (the number of calories one burns at rest) three-fold. Recipes in Dr. Chilton's book have been helpful in our meal planning over time as well.

The question for me is why I would want to live a long life if I am starving a good part of the time. I'd rather be full. I know this because I love to eat! I actually have much experience that contrasts the "starving" model with a "full" model, having been Queen of Diets in my younger years. Some of the diets were self-fashioned such as eating a muffin for breakfast, two or three of the red and white peppermint hard candies (which I would smash with a pair of scissors or other handy hard object to make the pieces last longer) over the course of the day, and a modest dinner with no dessert. I also tried one of the popular diet plans that sells you specific foods and endured periods when I just plain ignored the stomach growling. In contrast, Dr. Chilton's book will help you:

- Reduce calories
- Exercise to fight inflammation
- Add fiber in your diet and recipes
- Switch to Omega 3 fats in certain fish; one serving a day results in a 35 percent reduction in fatal heart disease.
- Increase resveratrol and polyphenols found in fruits and vegetables such as blueberries, cranberries, raspberries, broccoli, and plums–and red wine.

If you prefer, you can also search for book material online. We did that to print out a list of the fiber content in foods. The list now hangs on our refrigerator for quick reference.

Laugh Lines

A woman is sipping a glass of wine while sitting on the patio with her husband and she says, "I love you so much, I don't know how I could ever live without you!" Her husband asks, "Is that you or the wine talking?" She replies, "It's me . . . talking to the wine."

Lifestyle

Both Buettner's and Ward-Baker's research highlighted studies that reinforce a healthy physical lifestyle as a key ingredient to longevity. Suffice it to say that not smoking is a must, and exercise is key for not only physical health, but also mental and emotional health. Studies such as the FINE (Finland, Italy, and the Netherlands Elderly) directly link cardiovascular health with brain function. Within the exercise realm, walking and weight bearing exercise are king and queen, and diets low in fat, sugar, and salt, but packed with fiber and antioxidants protect against cancer, heart disease, and stroke. Again, this is common sense, but worth repeating.

Measurements Work

Working in the corporate world, I was steeped in measurement systems of all sorts, including the various quality measurements that have evolved from the Malcolm Baldrige days, such as "Six Sigma" or "the balanced scorecard." I was convinced that I could measure anything, regardless of how elusive the task might have seemed. I also understood that what gets measured gets attention. I still believe that that concept holds true.

Today, I like to measure my own behavior. I wear a pedometer to measure and track my steps, looking to achieve an average of 10,000 steps a day. I attempt to get my seven to eight hours of sleep each night. I count my sets and reps when lifting weights in the gym a minimum of twice a week, even if that means I drive forty-five minutes each way, as I do when in Maine. I make sure to have an annual physical that measures my vital signs and track my progress over time. Measurements are my connection to how I'm doing lately. If you haven't already started to measure your physical health beyond stepping on the scales occasionally, I highly recommend you start. Measuring the things that cause weight gain or loss versus just your weight on the scales will help you focus on the right things. Frankly, I rarely weigh myself on the scales.

Wisdom from the Ages

Lastly, let me just highlight some of the studies that perhaps some of you have been exposed to over time. Here are what two of the groups who have a high percentage of "engaged" centenarians recommend:

- The Seventh Day Adventists in Utah avoid alcohol, caffeine, and tobacco. They tend to live an average of eight years longer than the typical American.
- In Okinawa, a study of centenarians has been performed jointly by the United States National Institute for Health and Japan's Ministry of Health (since 1976). Centenarians there get plenty of exercise, both physical and mental. Their diets are low in fat and salt, and packed with fiber and antioxidants that protect against cancer, heart disease, and stroke. They consume more soy than an average American or Chinese person. They eat until they are 80 percent satisfied.

So will eating less improve longevity–or will it just seem that we live longer? In the 1930s, scientists found that underfed rodents lived 40 percent longer than well-fed counterparts. More recently, Dr. David Sinclair at Harvard found that fewer calories translate to lower blood pressure, glucose, and cholesterol levels. At the University of Wisconsin, gerontologist Richard Weindruch studies deprivation in monkeys and believes that less body fat protects against a range of ills. Apparently, starving the body puts it under mild, constant stress, priming it to resist more severe stresses that make cells age.

Yet another study released recently by the American Academy of Neurology followed 1,233 people age 70-90 in Olmsted County, Minnesota. The research found that the "odds of having mild cognitive impairment more than doubled in the highest calorie group (more than 2,143 daily) versus the lower calorie group (600-1,526 daily)." Thus, memory loss may be yet another good reason to limit sugar and eat healthful meals. My husband likes to point out that rarely will you see an obese person who has achieved a long life. However, eating the fiber-rich diet mentioned earlier will keep you lean as well as feeling full, our personal preference.

So we know that overeating is not good for us; why don't we act on that knowledge? When we get up in the morning, do we ever think about what we're going to do to bring us more balance or a healthier lifestyle? More importantly, is there some purpose within us that requires that we do that, a positive motivator?

The Power of Touch

Before we leave the discussion on physical well being, I want to mention one last aspect of our physical health: the power of touch. I know of three divorced men who have regular massages as their cure for lack of another's touch. We can even see the behavior of touch alive in the animal kingdom when a mare, for example, nuzzles her colt, or a chimpanzee grooms her baby. Then too, I so vividly remember during my mother's last days, how much she enjoyed being touched—even our rubbing her forehead as she lay in bed was a great comfort. Touch is a necessary sense we all need to give and get.

One wonderful freedom of age is that we can touch people without fear of a harassment suit (I think) or fear that it will lead to other things. It is fine for me, even normal, to hug a female or male friend. It's a greeting, in fact. Often even with strangers, I will bypass the traditional handshake and "go for the gold."

In our town in Maine, there is a seventy-something man whose hugging technique is unparalleled. Women seek him out, but he hugs both genders when they let him. In fact, I've told him that he should give lessons, which his wife says is "not going to happen"! Yet how many of us shy away from the touch a sincere hug can offer?

From my earlier working days in New York, I recall an incident with one of my directors who was quite a bit older than I was; he hugged me as we met instead of offering a handshake, and I was mortified. In retrospect, I'm guessing that he grew up with family members for whom hugging was the norm. It was not so in my family. I am not recommending that we all start hugging at work, especially with the potential harassment claims that would arise in today's business environment. However, I now feel free to make up for lost time. I'll hug anyone within arms' reach, and when my children are around, I've been known to hug them every time they enter the room. Lucky for me, they've gotten used to it.

"WE NEED FOUR HUGS A DAY FOR SURVIVAL. WE
NEED EIGHT HUGS A DAY FOR MAINTENANCE. WE
NEED TWELVE HUGS A DAY FOR GROWTH."
VIRGINIA SATIR, FAMILY THERAPIST

Laugh Lines

A husband and wife came for counseling after twenty years of marriage. When asked what the problem was, the wife went into a passionate, painful tirade listing every problem they had ever had since they had been married.

She went on and on and on: neglect, lack of intimacy, emptiness, loneliness, feeling unloved and unlovable – an entire laundry list of unmet needs she had endured over the course of their marriage.

Finally, after allowing this to go on for a sufficient length of time, the therapist got up, walked around the desk and, after asking the wife to stand, embraced and kissed her passionately as her husband watched with a raised eyebrow. The woman shut up and quietly sat down as though in a daze.

The therapist turned to the husband and said, "This is what your wife needs at least three times a week. Can you do this?"

The husband thought a moment and replied, "Well, I can drop her off here on Mondays and Wednesdays, but on Fridays, I fish!"

8

SOCIAL NETWORKING

"NO MAN IS POOR WHO HAS FRIENDS."
GEORGE BAILEY IN *IT'S A WONDERFUL LIFE*

Building Positive Relationships

In a gym my husband and I used to frequent, there was a sign posted that asserted that the three big things in life were exercise, nutrition, and social contact. Somehow, I hadn't thought of "social contact" as that important to my long-term health. I am delighted because as an extrovert, I've always loved being around others. Yet, the concept is even more important for those of us who prefer to be alone.

In a ten-year study at the MacArthur Foundation, utilizing data drawn from 7,000 U.S. adults in midlife, Carol Ryff, a scholar in the foundation's Interdisciplinary Network on Successful Midlife Development, says, "The quality of social relationships is a powerful predictor of how long one lives, the incidence of illness, and recovery rates from illness."

Buettner's "Blue Zones" findings clearly support the importance of having a strong social circle. He quotes a number of longitudinal studies that stress the importance of social connectedness in longevity. He advises that we should identify the people in our lives that "support healthy habits," challenge us mentally, and can be counted on in time of need. He warns us to be likeable and work at creating time together. The latter does take some thought and planning, but certainly carries rich rewards.

Although it is difficult for researchers to measure the impact of social relationships due to the multiple factors at play, it is clear that social involvement helps fight depression—which is common among those who withdraw from friends, family, and community. Social isolation is a strong risk factor for health problems and early death.

Those of you who volunteer in the schools reading to children may be interested in the study done by The Johns Hopkins Center on Aging and Health. The study looked at the Experience Corps program which places volunteers aged 59-86 in public elementary schools for fifteen hours a week. Not only did the academic outcomes of the children improve, but also the physical, cognitive, and social outcomes of volunteers.

Dr. Daniel Goleman at Harvard, who has done a lot of work with the concept of emotional intelligence, has also written a book on social intelligence which he calls a "revolutionary new science of human relationships." If you're interested in the subject and want to work the brain, you will enjoy his book.

On a lighter note, at a Duke Integrative Medicine Health Symposium I attended, the keynote speaker said that researchers have found that men who are married are healthier and happier. Of course, she added that women with pets are healthier and happier. Sorry, men.

In 1982, a friend sent me a *Newsweek* article written by Professor Elliot Engel, who was teaching at North Carolina State University at the time. The article asks the question, "Do you need a bosom to have a buddy?" He suggests that "the days of the mythic male friendship went out with the Greeks and can hardly be expected to flourish in modern America." He goes on to say, "If men would begin to personalize the concept of brotherhood by seeking more fraternal bonds with other men, they would find their freedom of expression and indeed their happiness greatly enhanced."

Recognizing that men seek bonds and display them in different ways than women do, I find this subject somewhat comical. I can return from a luncheon or social gathering with women having amassed numerous interesting (at least to me) stories regarding people's lives. My husband, on the other hand, can play tennis, hike, or soak in the hot tub with other men and remember very little about what was said. Phone conversations perhaps illustrate our gender differences even further. I may carry on for three minutes to his responses of "yes" or "no." Social interactions certainly do vary.

Redefining "Friend"

In one of my classes recently, we spent some time pondering the thought that often older people feel that they have outlived their friends, which can send some into depression or simply wishing that they too would "go." We had a lively discussion about the need to redefine our network of friends over time to purposefully include people of all ages.

This may have been easier in the past when generations of families lived together or in close-by circumstances. Today, this could require a little creative thought and social engineering. With families in the United States and indeed the world separated by distance, we have the good fortune of technologies such as the phone, Internet, and electronic "face time" to keep family members of all ages in touch. While working-age adults may be busy, often it is the younger grandchildren that most enjoy a conversation or virtual visit from a grandparent.

Then too, we have the opportunity to befriend a non-family member from a later generation through mentoring activities, schooling, and a variety of volunteering efforts. There is no lack of need in communities for more positive interaction between the ages. It simply requires that we decide what interests us, and find a way to share with others willing to be involved.

And lastly, a University of Michigan study found that the biggest effect on well being comes from the size of a retiree's social network. It outweighs even health and money. The study says that those of us with sixteen good pals are, on average, far more satisfied with life than those with ten friends or fewer. Right away, on reading this, I'm starting to count on my fingers how many good friends I have . . . uh, and what is a "good friend"? I think more research is required on this one.

9

EMOTIONAL LITERACY

"The heart has reason which reason
cannot understand."
Blaise Pascal

Let's consider that we define "emotional literacy" as "staying in touch with your feelings and managing them for a positive outcome." Think about your Life Balance Chart. If you are anything like me, your emotional growth was in need of some repair. Joe Gauld, who wrote *Character First* and is well known in character education circles, maintains that America has become "emotionally illiterate." Is it possible that our feelings are so hardened by the media and other input that we simply can't feel anymore?

The Study of Emotional Intelligence

Emotional Intelligence–EQ–is a relatively recent behavioral model, which rose to prominence with Daniel Goleman's 1995 book, *Emotional Intelligence*. He says he wrote the book due to what he perceived as a rise in human aggression and depression. The Emotional Intelligence theory was originally developed during the '70s and '80s by the work and writings of psychologists Howard Gardner

(Harvard), Peter Salovey (Yale), and John Mayer (New Hampshire).

These early investigations maintained that Emotional Intelligence is increasingly relevant to organizational development and to the development of people, because the EQ principles provide a new way to understand and assess people's behaviors, management styles, attitudes, interpersonal skills, and potential. Emotional Intelligence is an important consideration in human resources planning, job profiling, recruitment interviewing and selection, management development, customer relations, customer service, and more.

The EQ concept argues that the Intelligence Quotient (IQ), or conventional intelligence, is too narrow; there are wider areas of emotional intelligence that dictate and enable how successful we are. Success requires more than IQ, which has tended to be the traditional measure of intelligence, ignoring essential behavioral and character elements. We've all met people who are academically brilliant yet socially and interpersonally inept. And we know that a high IQ rating does not automatically equate to success.

Goleman identified the five "domains" of EQ as:

1. Knowing your emotions
2. Managing your own emotions
3. Motivating yourself
4. Recognizing and understanding other people's emotions
5. Managing relationships (and the emotions of others)

Per Mayer, people with higher emotional intelligence are likely to have better social support and fewer problematic interactions with others. They are less likely to abuse drugs and alcohol, more satisfied with their social networks—and they appear to receive more social support. Finally, they are seemingly more successful at avoiding interpersonal arguments and fights.

Most importantly, research indicates that the skills of emotional intelligence can be learned at any age.

Worry and Stress

Dr. Nancy Gordon, who has a Ph.D. in Pyscho-Neuro-Immunology (the study of the mind's impact on the body's immune system), is a wellness consultant, author, and Olympic swim team coach. She is a fan of meditation, visualization, and positive self talk. She gives the negative example of what happened in the United States following 9/11 when sickness in the country drastically increased. Our thoughts were literally making us sick! And today, uncertainty, lack of hope, and fears have given rise to "occupations" and violence.

Dr. Gordon believes that positive affirmations, positive beliefs, and passion make anything possible. She offers a technique for worry or stress: replace those thoughts with the question, "What am I grateful for right now? Just breathe in and out and think thoughts of gratitude . . . say it, feel it, visualize it." When we are positive, our cells are storing energy. When we are negative, it literally sucks the life out of us. Recall our examples in nature of the four seasons and how the trees in winter, their most stressful period, are using that time to restore their energy. Let's learn that lesson from nature.

Something that saps our emotions and takes away our ability to even focus on emotions, is stress—or the act of worrying. Webster says that stress is "a constraining force or influence . . . a physical, chemical, or emotional factor that causes bodily or mental tension and may be a factor in disease causation." It says that worry means to "choke or strangle . . . to feel or experience concern or anxiety."

In Matthew 6:25 to 6:34 of the Life Application Study Bible, we see some reasons not to worry:

- The same God who created life in you can be trusted with the details of your life.
- Worrying about the future hampers your efforts for today.
- Worrying is more harmful than helpful.
- There are real challenges God wants us to pursue, and worrying keeps us from them.
- Living one day at a time keeps us from being consumed with worry.

A second area to consider under emotional growth is our handling of stress. A study from the University of California confirmed what we knew all along: stress really does age people. When researchers studied women with chronically ill children, they found that these women had shorter telomeres than other women of the same age who weren't dealing with chronically ill children. Telomeres are the tiny caps on cells' chromosomes that govern cell regeneration. When the telomeres get too short, the cell stops dividing and eventually dies, causing aging. According to Judy Moskowitz, Ph.D., a psychologist at UCSF who worked on the study, "These telomeres are one of the few biological markers of aging we have."

In 2006, researchers reporting in the journal *Nature Medicine* were able to "pinpoint beta-2 receptors for adrenaline—the stress hormone—on actual tumor cells, leaving no question that stress was advancing cancer." According to Lorenzo Cohen, Ph.D., the director of MD Anderson's integrative medicine program, tumors grew 275 percent more in stressed test mice compared with non-stressed mice. They believe that these findings relate also to humans. There is also a well-established connection between stress and heart disease and the immune function in general.

Thomas Perls, M.D., an associate professor of medicine at Boston University and the Director of the New England Centenarian Project, said of a nationwide study of 1,500 people over the age of 100 and their children, "It isn't the amount of stress that matters, but how you manage it."

Think back to your teenage years. What stressed you then? For me, it might have been those blasted pimples that always seemed to pop out when I was anticipating a big date. How about the thirties and forties? I can assure you that at that point, my acne issues were far from my thoughts. Raising my children, finding nurturing babysitters, and keeping my family together trumped all. How about now? What are your top three current stressors? Someone recently told me they were "family, money, and family asking for money"! The point is that stressors and worries change significantly over time—which begs the question, "Why would we stress at all about things that are sure to seem insignificant at a later date in time?"

Stress Reducers

There are many who believe in the power of meditation and breathing to reduce stress. Healing Hearts, founded by Mimi Guarneri, M.D., teaches lifestyle change through such things as meditation, yoga, music therapy, nutrition, and exercise. Different strategies work for different people because stress reducers are individual things. Think about some of the stress reducers you employ over time that have helped you.

There are numerous studies and articles that highlight things people have done to reduce stress in their lives. In the July/August 2005 issue of AARP's magazine, the writers talked about some of the most common:

Work

Researchers have found that passionately engaging in work helps reduce stress, as well as the risk of depression, according to the *Journal of Humanistic Psychology*. Work that is flexible can negate the stressful effects of long hours, according to research from the University of Arkansas. We're speaking of work that is so meaningful that it becomes a calling far beyond the satisfaction of a nine-to-five job—regardless of the hours.

Exercise

Multiple studies from the University of Colorado have shown that physiological responses to stress from the brain, hormonal system, and immune system are moderated by regular exercise. Exercise reduces anxiety, releases tension, and spurs the brain to pump out endorphins, chemicals that create a sense of well being. Research suggests that if you do nothing else, walk for forty-five minutes, three days a week.

Close Friendships

Though loneliness has been linked to susceptibility to stress, depression, loss of cognitive ability, and other ills, friendships seem especially protective for women. Shelley

Taylor, a researcher at the University of California, has found that most women deal with stress by relying on long chats and talking through troubles with one another. Men are more likely to go into "fight or flight" mode, whereas women typically "tend and befriend." Although both males and females produce the soothing hormone oxytocin under stress, estrogen tends to enhance the hormone, while testosterone inhibits it. When oxytocin levels are high, people are calmer, more social, and less anxious. Friendships not only help fight stress, but also may partially explain why women tend to outlive men.

Music
While learning new things has been proven to beat stress, music has a special ability to calm people. Decades of research have shown that listening to music can lower blood pressure and heart rate. A study at the Mind-Body Wellness Center in Pennsylvania also found that playing music can significantly reduce stress.

Prayer
According to the *Journal of Health Psychology*, researchers know that among older people, spirituality, which covers not only faith and prayer, but also the close-knit support of religious communities, significantly lowers stress and improves the chances of recovering from serious illness.

A Sense of Humor
According to research from Western Illinois University, people who have the ability to make jokes tend to be more secure and confident in their interactions, less lonely, and more likely to see the stress in their lives as lower than those who aren't able to joke. Norman Cousins helped

pioneer "laugh therapy," as well as the medical discipline of psycho-neuro-immunology. He and other researchers have discovered that laughter and joy boosted immune functions to defend the body against infections and cancer.

Other stress reducers include thinking in a positive fashion and surrounding yourself with others who do so—and spending as much time as possible doing the things you love. As my daughter often says, "No worries," a phrase she picked up while living in Australia.

Finally, sometimes it is helpful to do a daily mental dump. I like to do that by sending an e-mail to someone about the issues of the day. I also am a fan of journals where I can just write down whatever I feel each day. The theory is that by writing things down, you can more easily release them from their grasp on you. It seems to work for many people.

And, my personal favorite—learning to say "no" to extra projects for which you have neither the time nor energy to complete. I am still working on this one!

The Worry Bag

I am someone who believes that everything happens for a reason, and if we are open to receiving messages, we will see them. Last spring, I was on the treadmill at the gym chatting with two of my friends, and the conversation changed from the beautiful spring weather to Easter and then to Lent and the Catholic tradition of giving up things for Lent. Those of you who are women can relate to such conversations. One of the women said that she had a friend who decided to give up worrying for Lent. Apparently, the friend got a shoebox, cut a hole in the top, and every time she felt like worrying, she wrote the worry on a piece of paper and put it in the box, defying herself to think about it any longer. After Easter, she took out the box, dumped out the worries, and realized that none of the worries had come to pass; so what really is the point of worrying? Mark Twain is credited with saying, "I am now an old man and have known many troubles, but most of them never happened."

I have created my own "worry bag" and I must say that there is something to the practice of consciously writing down a worry and throwing it into the bag. Periodically, I check out my collection, and I too have found that few of the entries evolve into anything beyond an anxious thought.

Laugh Lines

A woman in a supermarket is following a grandfather and his misbehaving three-year-old grandson. It's obvious to her that he has his hands full with the child screaming for sweets in the candy aisle and for fruit, cereal, and pop in the other aisles. Meanwhile, Granddad is working his way around, saying in a controlled voice, "Easy, William, we won't be long. Easy, boy."

At the checkout, the little terror is throwing items out of the cart and the granddad says again in a controlled voice, "William, William, relax, buddy, don't get upset. We'll be home in five minutes."

Very impressed, the woman goes outside where the grandfather is loading his groceries and the boy into the car. She said to the elderly gentleman, "It's none of my business, but you were amazing in there. That whole time, you kept your composure. No matter how loud and disruptive he got, you just calmly kept saying that things would be okay. William is very lucky to have you as his grandpa."

"Thanks," said the grandfather, "but I'm William. The little angel's name is Kevin."

10

SPIRITUAL GROWTH

"Faith consists in believing when it is beyond
the power of reason to believe."
Voltaire

Messages are Everywhere

Seven years ago, my husband Warren and I moved to
the "Bible Belt" in the Carolinas. As a Catholic, I had studied religious concepts in catechisms, but I had never owned
a Bible. Believing that I was in this region for a reason, I
decided it was time to learn something about the Bible, so
I bought one and joined a study group. Through the group,
I learned that there are ways to better connect with God
than I had regularly practiced in the past:

1. Read the Bible.
2. Go to church.
3. Live life with awareness.
4. Pray.

One night, I was sitting on the couch reading the Bible,
and frankly, I was not understanding a word and wondering how it could possibly foster a better connection to
God.

I decided to call it a night and headed to the bathroom

to relieve myself. Of course, I saw that both the lid and the seat of the toilet were in the upright position. I pulled the top one down and noticed on the bottom of the second one, what I thought was the word "Church" . . . no kidding! I hurried back to the couch and returned with my glasses to get a better look. Sure enough, on the bottom of the toilet seat cover I saw the word "Church."

I was then motivated to run around the house and look at the other toilets, thinking that maybe the word would disappear while I was wandering. The upstairs toilet has the word "Bemis" on it, and the third one had nothing. I returned to the first toilet and the word "Church" was still there. I decided that I'd better call my friend who had offered to take me to church in the area, and that I probably should do it soon! Number two on my list of ways to connect with God was now number one.

I made the call, and off I went to a Baptist church the next Sunday. I really liked it; the music was incredible. Then, one Sunday, the minister asked everybody who had been "saved" to raise their hands. Given that I didn't have a clue what that meant, I didn't raise my hand. I was probably the only one in the church who didn't raise his or her hand, and of course, I felt people looking at me. I decided that perhaps being a Baptist wasn't my thing.

The next week, I went to an Episcopalian church. Successive weeks found me at a Presbyterian church, a Catholic church, and a Methodist church. Another friend said I should try the Lutheran church nearby and that she would meet me there.

I finally made it to the Lutheran church and felt quite comfortable, other than feeling obligated to stand up and introduce myself for several weeks as a guest, which seemed like a bit of an overkill for the audience–but, I was trying to follow the rules. I did like the openness there and their focus on growth. I signed up for a class that promised to tell me something about my "spiritual gifts" and was hooked. I now call myself a "Lutheran," and it feels rather liberating to have chosen a denomination that supports me and fosters my growth, rather than simply practicing my childhood orientation.

For those of you who have stepped away from religious affiliations over time and are interested in spiritual growth, I highly recommend you look around to find a church or spiritual community that suits you and your lifestyle today. It is not only a fun experience to see how different religions "celebrate," but also an opportunity to meet some wonderful people and to grow both emotionally and spiritually in the process.

Laugh Lines

An elderly couple would constantly argue about everything. The woman often ended the arguments by stating vociferously, "I'll dance on your grave!" Well, sure enough, the man died first. His last request was that he be buried at sea.

The Case for A Spiritual Community

In Buettner's *The Blue Zones*, one of the common denominators of the centenarians he studied was simply: "Belong (participate in a spiritual community)." Apparently healthy centenarians in Buettner's research have faith.

Buettner cited two other studies that agree with his own. In one, researchers for the *Journal of Health and Social Behavior* followed 3,617 people for seven and a half years and found that those who attended religious services at least once a month reduced their risk of death by about a third. As a group, the attendees had a longer life expectancy, with an impact about as great as that of moderate physical activity. In the National Institute of Health Adventist Health Study, researchers followed more than 34,000 people over a period of twelve years and found that those who went to church services frequently were 20 percent less likely to die at any given age and that they had lower rates of cardiovascular disease, depression, stress, and suicide; their immune systems just seemed to work better.

Although I personally am a Christian, for our collective thought process I would not propose that there is a favored religion. Remember that we are talking about a "spiritual community," not necessarily a religious organization.

Defining Spirituality

An unknown author wrote: "Religion is for those people who are afraid they'll go to hell and spirituality is for those who have already been there."

I suggest that the quest for one's unique potential constitutes a spiritual journey. A Tibetan writer, Djwhal Kahul, has said, "Everything is spiritual which tends toward understanding, toward kindness . . . and leads man to a fuller expression of his divine potential."

Faith is a belief in a higher power, a universal order, or some force behind creation. Sometimes, we are lucky enough to see that power at work through survival of human beings under exceptional circumstances. A friend of ours who had brain cancer was an amazing example of that. It started with his positive attitude, even as his doctors and insurance company were saying that rehab was not available to him because it was a waste of money. His family decided to bring him home and treat him there instead. He was convinced that the power of prayer improved his quality of life and gave him the strength to fight all odds and extend his life another two years while enjoying some of his favorite activities, such as golf, once again.

Author Craig Barnes, who wrote *When God Interrupts,* says spirituality is not a thing like nature, but more an attitude of gratitude and honoring our creator by becoming who you are. He goes on to say that being "too focused on faith is like trying to improve our vision by taking off our glasses and looking at them. The point is to look through them, not at them." Faith isn't an external thing; it is part of who we are.

As we head into our next chapter pondering our sense of purpose, we will think of spirituality as the basic premise: "Who are you?" and "Who are you becoming?" It is a point of reference that permeates everything we do.

Meditation . . . Again

When studying several life components in our Life Balance exercise, meditation is often mentioned as a way to help us enhance capabilities such as spiritual growth. Believe it or not, there is a Meditation Society of America that has documented 108 meditation techniques. You'll be happy to know that I will not go over all of those. However, three quotes from the Society in their "words of wisdom" seem relevant:

- "If at first you don't succeed, that's what was supposed to happen."
- "Empty your mind of negativity and the universe will fill it with love, wisdom, and bliss."
- "Great wealth will not bring you peace. The minute you get it, you start worrying you will lose it. Real peace is the greatest pleasure."

The Meditation Society explains the stages of going into meditation. It starts with the "normal mind" which is bombarded by thoughts that flit in and out all day long. When we decide to meditate, we enter a state called the "concentrating mind." We pick a subject to focus on, such as love. However, for most of us, the mind continues to distract us with thoughts of love that then migrate to love of something like chocolate. Then we drift to thoughts of going to a store to get some, and then selecting the chocolate from the many choices, and so on. The mind is still very active in this stage.

The next stage, referred to as the "meditating mind," is one in which we continue to focus on love, but it takes on new forms such as fatherly love, unconditional love, love of country, puppy love, and so on. The Society speaks of Albert Einstein who felt that "everything in the universe is relative to everything else," and that "ultimately your meditation on love will connect you to everything."

The final stage, "contemplating mind," is the ultimate state of consciousness. We become "conscious of the cosmos and know ourselves to be part of it and realize our unity with all of it."

The Society has specific meditation techniques for emotional, intellectual, physical, and spiritual activities. If you have not tried meditation and are willing to experiment with it, seek a technique that will work for you, and give it a try. I don't think you'll be disappointed. I find that meditation can't be done on an annual basis (I've tried that). It requires practice and regular use if you expect to experience the full benefit of it. However, it is worthwhile, and it's something you can do anytime, anywhere.

The Preferred State

We have seen that although we start life in a balanced fashion, many of us get distracted along the way with behaviors that pull us away from our preferred states. Thank goodness we arrive in midlife with things to adjust and work on to keep us in a growth mode. Then too, during our journey in life we have shaped ourselves into the amazing people we are today, each of us different from every other person on earth who has lived or is living now. With those thoughts in mind, it is time to turn to your sense of purpose.

Laugh Lines

Paddy was driving down the street in a sweat because he had an important meeting and couldn't find a parking place. Looking up to heaven he said, "Lord, take pity on me. If you find me a parking place, I'll go to Mass every Sunday for the rest of me life and give up me Irish whiskey for Lent!"

Miraculously, a parking place appeared. Paddy looked up again and said, "Never mind, Lord, I found one."

11

STEP THREE:
A BROADER, DEEPER SENSE OF PURPOSE
Living through Principles

"The two most important days in your life are the day you were born, and the day you find out why."
Mark Twain

We have now positioned ourselves for change, discovered new things about ourselves, and explored some opportunities for additional growth through the concept of life-long learning. In this chapter, we will look at the importance of sense of purpose and construct a sense of purpose that is relevant for each of us.

Stephen Covey used the term "leading principle-centered lives" to describe men and women of character who work with competence on farms on the basis of natural principles they built into their lives. Farming is such a great metaphor for so many things. There are no "quick fixes" in farming. One must prepare the ground, plant the seed, cultivate it, weed it, water it, and gradually nurture growth to full maturity. Only then, can we harvest the goods . . . when they are ready.

Covey calls this the "Laws of the Farm." And so it is with principles, which run far deeper than rules. Think about rules versus principles. I remember as a parent learning about living by principles the hard way. Warren and I had rules we expected the kids to live by: don't fight with each other; do your homework; don't leave your clothes on the floor, etc. And as fast as we came up with the rules which ran all the way down the refrigerator on a never-ending list, the kids would do something that required yet another rule. Once we dug deeper, we realized that what we really needed was to establish–and to model–principles that no one could bypass. They needed to be clear, deep, and far-reaching. Two principles that made sense to us were honesty and responsibility.

Think of some principles in your life that you believe are at your core, perhaps things you learned as a child. Before looking ahead, write down a few. Toss out some of them, and add some additional ones.

Now let's open your minds a bit further with an exercise on personal ideals–that is, things that are important to you in life. Looking at the list below, pick your five most critical ideals. If you want to add another ideal that doesn't appear on the list, but is of high importance to you, please do so. List the ideals in order of preference where number one is your primary ideal and so forth through number five:

Collaborating with others	Being loyal
Being well known	Serving others
Spending time with family and friends	Being creative
Being part of something	Maintaining physical fitness
Influencing others	Gaining new knowledge
Challenging myself	Being independent
Being spiritually grounded	Having time freedom
Advancing my career or life work	Being self motivated
Having security	Having power
Making my own decisions	Having low stress
Having major accomplishments	Overcoming obstacles
Being active in the community	Having authority
Being competitive	Using new skills

There was a time in my life, as I found my direction in transition, when I carried my list of ideals with me to maintain my integrity and to keep me pointed in the right direction. I made decisions with the list in mind. Today, I periodically review and update my list as my life situations change. For example, during my corporate years, "being competitive" and "having power" were on my list. They no longer make the cut. Good thing given my performance on the tennis court these days!

Thinking about your ideals, as well as evaluating results from your life balance exercise and the Keirsey Temperament Sorter, can give you insight into your sense of purpose, because again, sense of purpose is at our core, deep within us; it is who we are meant to be.

A Broader View

The dissertation for my Ph.D. addressed a sense of purpose for my study participants–before and after a challenging growth process over a period of one to three years. Participants considered the questions "Who am I?" and "Who am I becoming?" Some examples are as follows:

Sense of Purpose Before and After

Before: Good wife, good mother, good professor
After: Help people in my area of expertise.

Before: Cloudy, not defined.
After: Live a life that is meaningful to me, that involves my family, people I'm close to, the ideals I hold to be

most important, but with more love, humor, and compassion.

Before: Raising the family
After: Find out what makes me tick, what I like to do, and how I can help others.

Before: Being a good mother
After: Being a good person

Over time, responses generally began to show more introspection and more consideration of the participants' value to others. They also touched on deep-seated needs to leave a legacy or to fulfill some higher purpose.

Sense of purpose is the same. I used to think my sense of purpose was to get an "A" in school, to find a job, to become a parent, or to fulfill some such role or mission. Sense of purpose was like a short-term goal to me. I now know that my sense of purpose is much broader than any one or all of those things. It is my core in life; it is what is at my center. It is almost like a message from my conscience leading me in a direction, but without a clear destination per se, although I'm always on the lookout. It feels like I have been prepared to do something all my life.

It is what Ward-Baker thinks of as "Internally Guided Forward" or what Buettner calls "Purpose Now." In its most simple form, it's what gets you out of bed in the morning. Buettner even supposes that, "The strong sense of purpose possessed by older Okinawans may act as a buffer against stress and help reduce their chances of suffering from Alzheimer's disease, arthritis and stroke."

In Dr. Perls's studies of centenarians in the Boston area, the participants' sense of purpose could be as basic as knowing that the family depended on them to bring cookies to family celebrations each year. *The Blue Zones* notes a study done by Dr. Robert Butler and others led by the National Institute of Health. It was an eleven-year study that followed "highly functioning people" between the ages of sixty-five and ninety-two and found that individuals who expressed a clear goal in life lived longer and were sharper than those who did not. In addition, it was reported that immediately following December 31, 1999, demographers saw a spike in deaths among elders. These older people, in other words, may have willed themselves to stay alive into the new millennium. Once there, their will to live was gone. Clearly, their sense of purpose was date-timed, rather than focused on their larger contribution in life.

The Midlife Advantage

The American writer Madeleine L'Engle, who died at age eighty-eight, said, "The great thing about getting older is that you don't lose all the other ages you've been." One of the advantages of living into and through midlife is that we have a lot of history, experiences, influences, and clues to draw on to form our sense of purpose. I was able to articulate my own sense of purpose about sixteen years ago, and I am pretty clear that it is what it is. When I stray from it–and I do–I get lethargic, even sick or injured.

On the other hand, when I am in my "zone," it is almost like an out of body experience for me. Dr. Mihaly Csikszentmihalyi, mentioned in *The Blue Zones*, describes that experience as a "Zen-like state of total oneness with the activity at hand in which you feel fully immersed in what you're doing." He says, "It's characterized by a sense of freedom, enjoyment, fulfillment, and skill, and while you're in it, temporal concerns (time, food, etc.) are typically ignored. If you can identify the activity that gives you this sense of flow and make it the focus of your job or hobby, it can also become your sense of purpose."

This hits home with me every time I teach. I spend days updating my material with the latest knowledge I can find, and I easily lose track of time. I look forward to seeing my students every week and to the excitement of teaching the class. I mentioned earlier that I had recently attended a workshop focused on helping people find their spiritual gifts. In my case, I learned that my "demonstrated passions" were influencing, teaching, improving, and developing. I don't believe for a second that any of that is happenstance. I believe that it is all part of who I am supposed to become in life's plan.

Okay, so what is my sense of purpose crafted sixteen years ago and still very much alive in my life today? Simply put, I will "be the best I can be, help others do the same, and thus, leave the world a better place." I do not take credit for it, and I may have even piggy-backed on someone else's sense of purpose along the way, perhaps Joe Gauld's. Feel free to do the same if that works for you. At any rate, that is midlife leadership for me, and it is my credo for the rest of my life. Do I live it every day? Probably not, but I think I'm moving in the right direction. And hey, I have another fifty-four years left to get it right! Joe Gauld's son Malcolm said that Pablo Casals, a famous cellist, at age ninety-four, was once asked why he still practiced the cello six hours a day. He replied, "Because I think I am making progress!"

PABLO CASALS, A FAMOUS CELLIST, AT AGE NINETY-FOUR, WAS ONCE ASKED WHY HE STILL PRACTICED THE CELLO SIX HOURS A DAY. HE REPLIED, "BECAUSE I THINK I AM MAKING PROGRESS!"

Where and how to apply your sense of purpose is another story and something we will discuss in the next chapter as Step Four of our leadership development strategy in midlife: unique potential.

So we see that sense of purpose is what gets you up in the morning; it gives you a terrific sense of fulfillment, and you know it when you're in its "zone." In addition, it is broad in application and easy to articulate and focus on. Think about this: What if I want to just stay in bed in the morning? I can't do that, and believe me I have tried. My sense of purpose literally propels–okay, sometimes rolls me out of bed in the morning. Sort of annoying, huh? Then I have a healthy high fiber breakfast (part of being the best I can be) and start my day. My day always includes exercise of some sort, along with prayer, social connections, and intellectual challenges. I don't have a choice. If I want a quality life, I have to do these things to obtain and to maintain it. And how can I help anyone else, if I don't practice what I preach? I'll leave that effort to our politicians! To maintain my integrity, I for one, need to "walk the talk."

Craft Your Sense of Purpose

Take a minute to think about the principles by which you live, the ideals you have, and your own sense of purpose. How would you describe your sense of purpose today? Think BIG picture; this is not an exercise for wimps. Some examples from my last class included "to create beauty" (crafted by an artist), "to serve others" (crafted by a former nurse), and "to create joy" (crafted by a grandmother). As you can see, they don't have to be as long as mine; short is good and easy to remember.

With your broad sense of purpose in hand, you are ready to look at how you now can apply it to your life activities as your unique potential takes shape. If you were unable to craft a specific sense of purpose at this time, borrow mine, which probably fits for most of us and is broad enough to encompass your journey forward.

Laugh Lines

My friend Bill told me that he took his dad to the mall the other day to buy some new shoes. His dad is ninety-two. They decided to grab a bite to eat at the food court. Bill's dad seemed to be watching a teenager at the table next to them. The teenager had spiked hair; some spikes were green, while others were red, orange, or blue. Bill's dad kept staring at him. The teenager would glance his way and find him staring every time.

When the teenager had had enough, he sarcastically asked, "What's the matter, old man, never done anything wild in your life?"

Bill figured, knowing his dad, that he'd have a good response, and he did: "Yeah, I got drunk once and had relations with a peacock. I was just wondering if you were my son."

12

STEP FOUR:
PURSUIT OF UNIQUE POTENTIAL
The Self in Connection

"THE MAIN THING, OF COURSE, ALWAYS IS THE
FACT THAT THERE IS ONLY ONE OF YOU IN THE
WORLD, JUST ONE, AND IF THAT IS NOT FULFILLED
THEN SOMETHING HAS BEEN LOST. THERE'S A
LIVING POTENTIAL FOR EACH ONE OF US IF WE
CHOOSE TO TAKE IT."
MARTHA GRAHAM, AT AGE 96

Vocation

When we did the Life Balance exercise in an earlier chapter, we talked about there being an area of our lives beyond the intellectual, physical, social, emotional, and spiritual, called "vocation." Aristotle said, "Where talents and the needs of the world cross, therein lies your vocation." Vocation may or may not be what you've done for "work" in or out of your home. Regardless of the labeling we choose, midlife is the time to do something you love, something that seems right to you. I know of no true leaders in the world who were not driven by something within them that trumped bringing home a paycheck. However, it is also true that when you focus on a passion, the likelihood that the money will follow is high.

ARISTOTLE SAID, "WHERE TALENTS AND THE NEEDS OF THE WORLD CROSS, THEREIN LIES YOUR VOCATION."

One can arrive at a vocation in a number of ways. I remember reading a magazine that included an article about a woman who had lost her husband and son in a plane crash. She had been injured and had to use crutches to get around. After the tragedy, and as a result of her experience on crutches, she decided to start a business selling attractive, comfortable padded crutches made of a variety of fabrics. Anyone who has ever needed crutches can see that this was a stroke of brilliance. Crutches were ripe for change! She sold 100,000 crutches her first full year in business.

We most often think of vocation as "work," but a vocation–unlike the traditional connotation of work–can be paid or unpaid; it can certainly be volunteer work. It can be employment or a work of passion. Both count. I recently saw a bumper sticker that read, "Get involved. The world is run by those who show up!" Thus, vocation will tie in with our discussion of unique potential.

Let's assume that most of you have a sense of purpose defined. Perhaps others of you are still thinking about what is best for you. My sense of purpose, as mentioned earlier, is that I want to be the best I can be, help others do the same, and in that way, leave the world a better place. Borrow mine, if it fits. Now that we're out of bed and ready to go, the next question is how do we apply our sense of purpose? Who do we become over time?

The Self in Connection

A Biblical Interpretation

The Bible illustrates over and over how God takes what He created and uses it for its intended purpose. The story of Moses is a great example. Moses was tending a flock of sheep for his father-in-law when a voice coming from a burning bush told Moses to bring the Israelites out of Egypt. His response (Exodus 3:11) was, "Who am I that I should go to Pharaoh and bring the Israelites out of Egypt?"

Throughout Moses's life, he was at his finest and worst responding to conflicts around him. God didn't change who or what Moses was; He didn't give him new abilities and strengths. Instead, he took Moses's characteristics and molded them until they were suited for His purposes. Thus we see Moses's unique potential as he becomes a buffer between God and the people, and then leads the Israelites out of Egypt with the sea parted before them.

A Business Interpretation: Vision and Mission

Think of this another way: If I were a business owner, I might say that my sense of purpose is my "vision" and my unique potential is my "mission." Then, I'd develop my strategies to accomplish it all. For example, John F. Kennedy articulated the vision to "put a man on the moon." NASA's mission then focused on bringing the knowledge, resources, and people together to make that happen. Strategies must have included developing a profile for the ideal astronaut and a process for preparing those who would be chosen. Another strategy would certainly focus on developing the vehicle to get them there, and the list would go on from there.

A Character Interpretation

Still another way to look at unique potential is Joe Gauld's assertion that "people bring out the best in themselves by pursuing their unique potential." A unique potential is akin to an inner calling and reflects individual temperament, gifts, natural talents, dreams, aspirations, background, and traditions. It is the person in each of us waiting to be born from our unique amalgamation of background and experiences.

The Greek Interpretation

The Greek philosopher Socrates is credited with the phrase "Know thyself," which is inscribed on the main entrance to the Temple of Delphi. In classical Greek, "eudaimonia" was used as a term for the "highest human good." The aim of practical Greek philosophy was then to determine for each of us "what is it?" and "how can it be achieved?" Greek philosophy is often reduced to two simple credos: "Know thyself" (sense of purpose), and "Become who you are" (pursue unique potential).

Who Am I?

That sounds easy enough, but each of us has a unique way of defining who we are, often using roles or titles such as "mother" or "CEO." We often rely on "head thinking" as we sort through the answers, without taking advantage of our emotional feelings dictated by our hearts or what the conscience or spirit might be telling us. Do we live our lives, trusting this inner voice or attempt to control life through our strong will, our head thinking? If we're honest with ourselves, most of us choose the latter. What is an "inner voice" anyway? I happen to believe it's the Holy Spirit or my conscience, speaking for God. Some might say it's the soul speaking.

Although I can't claim perfection in the conscience area, I am the kind of person who has gone back into a store to report that the clerk forgot to charge me for a package of bottled water placed under the cart. I could never take an extra dollar in change when I know it is too much. I remember counseling one of my children in that regard. We had done some grocery shopping at a small store in our town, and when we got back to the car, I noticed that my son had taken a strawberry from the produce display. Both he and I remember my words to him as we went back to the store to pay for the strawberry, "A strawberry today, a stereo tomorrow." My honesty principle at work, I guess. And yes, I can and have ignored it when it wasn't convenient to listen. That is when my Irish Catholic guilt takes over my life. Not a pretty sight! Someone once told me that the real ultimate is Southern Baptist guilt. She said, "The kid, had he grown up a Southern Baptist, would have been so shamed by the strawberry incident, he might have hated himself for decades." No one can truthfully claim that religious organizations are perfect.

On a broader scale, there is something in our spirit that does seem to have the answers we seek. What I have found was that once I tuned in, usually because I was desperate and finally realized I didn't have all the answers, I began seeing clues around me. Have you ever encountered an inexplicable coincidence in your life? Perhaps something happened that seemed just too weird to be explained by reason and logic?

For example, my husband and I were driving back to Massachusetts from Maine when suddenly, on a particularly remote section of the road, our car had no acceleration and began to slow down. We came around a corner, and low and behold, the car stopped right in front of a gas station in the semi-wilderness. We were out of gas, even though the gauge told us the tank had plenty. It was fortuitous to be able to fill up right away, rather than walk for miles to get help.

Another example was how I landed my last corporate position in executive counseling, a new area for me. I was then in my Ph.D. program and needed to do an internship. Frankly, the thought of doing an "internship" somewhat baffled me at the time. An internship involves gaining supervised practical experience, which somehow I related to young adult college students. Apparently regardless of age, we all need "supervised practical experience" in a new field, which I was to learn shortly. At any rate, I thought my internship might involve teaching leadership or business administration classes at a college or university. I now can see that was "one-off" from the grand plan laid out for me by the One in charge.

During my search for the ideal internship, I received a phone call from a man who owns a small firm that helps executives and middle managers worldwide who are looking for a career change or other transition in their lives. I had actually worked with this firm as a client when I was looking for help with my own transition in corporate life some five years earlier. He asked if I would have lunch with him to "catch up," which I did. I left that luncheon with an internship which later morphed into one of the best jobs of my life over a six-year span. Was it happenstance, or was it part of a grand plan to prepare me for my next venture?

The concept of pursuing unique potential is played out in the movie "Pursuit of Happyness" starring Will Smith. It is a film based on the true story of Chris Gardner, a salesman who goes door-to-door selling bone density machines to doctors. His is a job that one could say was not his calling. One day, he passes the Dean Witter headquarters and notices that people coming out of the building are smiling and seemingly "happy." Smith's character wants to be happy as well. He finds out that these folks are stockbrokers and says to himself, "I'm good at math. I like dealing with people." Through his use of the Rubik's Cube, he also demonstrates his ability to use logic. And so, in this way, he looks at his life experience, he determines what he wants from life, and he evaluates the skills that would help him take his ideal next step. He is, as we say, in pursuit of unique potential–something he defines as "happiness." Given that Gardner went on to enjoy incredible success on Wall Street, the question we are left with is this: "Was Gardner's arrival in front of Dean Witter a coincidence?"

Carl Jung defines "synchronicity" as a "meaningful coincidence of two or more events where something other than the probability of chance is involved." I recognize synchronicity in my life all the time, and the more I see it, the more synchronicities appear. For example, my son, who was between jobs, was heavy on my mind as I visited my physical therapist after an accident. I wasn't really focused on what my therapist was saying until she started relating a recent experience she had facilitating a youth group, which was just what I needed to hear. I somehow knew then that my son would be fine. Shortly thereafter, he began teaching and working as a coach and mentor with young high school students.

An everyday example of synchronicity might be receiving a phone call from a loved one or friend at the exact moment you are thinking about them. This happens to me so often, it's eerie. I'm sure all of us, if we thought about it, could come up with more stories that give credence to "synchronicity."

Crafting Your Unique Potential

As we have stated earlier, unique potential is an individual thing. Some of us may never discover ours, but the point is that we continue to pursue it. There are no right or wrong answers. Each experience we, or our ancestors before us, have had in life helps shape our puzzle. A friend of mine who worked with me in telecommunications ended her career as an executive within what is now Verizon. She is married to a man who was the provost of a New England college. Every year, we exchanged Christmas letters. With few exceptions, she would mention that they were "spackling," meaning they were remodeling something in their home. It was a constant in their lives as careers happened, kids grew up, and houses came and went. Upon retirement, no surprise to me, she and her husband founded a company that buys large older homes and converts them into condos. Deep within them all along was a desire to build and reshape, a sense of purpose. They had taken that sense of purpose and crafted a business–unique potential in the making.

Another real life example of someone's pursuing unique potential involves a former client of mine who had always wanted to live in Hawaii. Although a man with considerable corporate experience, he aspired to becoming a minister and relished the time he spent at his church in various roles. He also loved boats and being on the water. To make a long story short, he went to seminary and became a minister, moved with his wife to Hawaii, leased a large boat, and began a new business performing funeral services at sea.

On a grander scale, Dr. Martin Luther King Jr. gave his life to pursue his unique potential. Mother Teresa certainly lived her unique potential. Some would say that Ronald Reagan followed an unlikely path to become one of the most honored Presidents and world leaders of our time. In all cases, their potential was planted at birth and shaped by life and circumstances.

Who Am I Becoming?

Remember that unique potential may not be a new profession or business. It is about finding a way to serve others. Some of us may not want to start a new business right now. However, all of us have within us an inner voice directing our next phase in life that is far beyond our pure "intellectual thinking." As Yogi Berra said, "When you come to a fork in the road, take it!" And for the skeptics in the group, even if you don't believe that you have a "unique potential," how can you go wrong with continual growth, being your best in all stages of life, and helping others do the same? As we grow, our focus shifts from ourselves to fulfilling our larger purpose in life. Exposure-growth-exposure-growth. It is the "Spiral of Change" at work, always digging down to our core.

How can you go wrong with continual growth, being your best in all stages of life, and helping others do the same?

Before we begin the process to set you on the path to discovering unique potential, I want to provide some caveats; once again, there are no quick fixes here. Consider the story I heard at the Hyde School of the man who found and watched a butterfly struggling to break out of its cocoon. After a while, the man decided to cut the cocoon to help the butterfly emerge and truncate the struggle. So what happens? The butterfly emerges and spends the rest of its short life crawling around with a swollen body and shriveled wings. It turns out that the struggle required for the butterfly to get through the tiny opening is nature's way of forcing fluid from the body of the butterfly into its wings, preparing it for flight. We can't rush nature or the "laws of the farm"!

Pursuing unique potential works the same way; it takes time. I am taking what evolves over our first fifty to eighty-something years of life and suggesting a method, one that has worked for me with hundreds of clients, to help you sift through your journey in a fulfilling way. What is new about the process is that I am packaging it in a way that should help you draw conclusions through your reading of this book. Therefore, you undoubtedly will need to take the information you think about and/or write, put it aside, and return to it again before reaching any final conclusions. I only wish that I could be there with you to hear your observations. Several things are certain:

- We each have a unique potential that can shape our life journey. Accept that as truth.

106

- It is clear that the United States is blessed with a plethora of folks who have extraordinary experiences and talents that cannot be denied, should not be taken for granted, and should be used to keep each of us at our best as well as help others reach their best over time.
- As we look at studies on centenarians, we cannot deny that there are extraordinary people in many corners of the world.
- To change the image of "seniors" from "old and unable," we need to get on with the task of creating the new vision of "movers and shakers," continuing to contribute to making the world a better place as we move into our centenarian years.

TO CHANGE THE IMAGE OF "SENIORS" FROM "OLD AND UNABLE," WE NEED TO GET ON WITH THE TASK OF CREATING THE NEW VISION OF "MOVERS AND SHAKERS," CONTINUING TO CONTRIBUTE TO MAKING THE WORLD A BETTER PLACE AS WE MOVE INTO OUR CENTENARIAN YEARS.

Making the world a better place sounds so lofty, doesn't it? I am reminded of the little boy on the beach who noticed during low tide that many of the starfish that had been washed up on shore were dying. He began throwing them back in the water one at a time. An older man came along and asked him what he was doing. The little boy responded that he was saving the starfish. The man then said, "But there are too many. You can't save all these starfish." The little boy picked up another starfish and threw it in the water commenting, "I just saved that one!"

Out with the Old

In order to help us reset our new vision, it would be helpful to have a label that stands out from the "seniors" and "old folks" of the past. Just as the label "Baby Boomers" facilitates our thinking of a section of our population, we too need a refreshed and vibrant image of who we are as a group. The new label needs to be one that depicts an engaged, enthusiastic, sharp and cutting edge kind of person like yourself. We will be "keen-agers"! In a search of synonyms for "keen" as the front end of our label, you would find such words as "deep, powerful, strong, profound, extreme, ardent, and lively." To me, any of those words renders a more positive image than the synonym for "senior" as "older and oldest," or the synonym for "old" as "ancient." Words have meanings, and it is time to redefine our group of mid-lifers with a word that we can relate to in a good way. The fact that "keen-ager" rhymes with "teenager" puts us in good company with those in our culture who are on a steep growth curve. If the term "keen-ager" also seems to have some relevance to my surname Keene, I will call it literary license.

A Keen-ager . . . Becoming Who You Are

One last caveat. For some of you, pursuing unique potential may go against what your ego would prefer. It will undoubtedly lead you to do things that are hard or that you'd prefer not to do. If you do choose the unique potential path, one thing is for sure: you will make a positive difference in your own life and the lives of those around you. Change and growth are always a bit of a struggle, yet the rewards are worth it. In this case, you are becoming who you are. How much better does that get?

OUT WITH THE OLD
FEATURING KELLY KEEN AND THE KEEN-AGERS

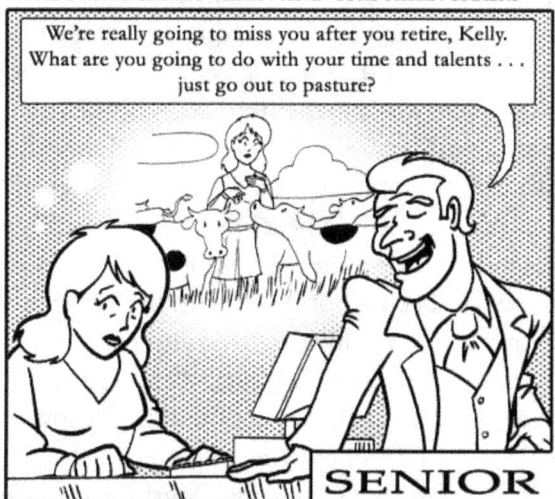

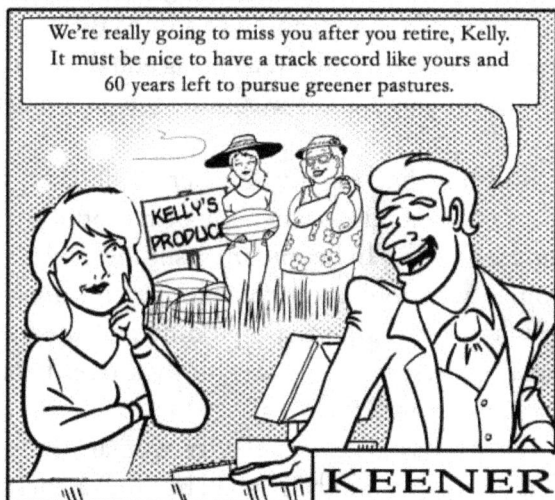

We're really going to miss you after you retire, Kelly. What are you going to do with your time and talents . . . just go out to pasture?

SENIOR

We're really going to miss you after you retire, Kelly. It must be nice to have a track record like yours and 60 years left to pursue greener pastures.

KELLY'S PRODUCE

KEENER

What Did Your Parents/Grandparents Love to Do?

We'll begin by preparing a template. For this exercise, you will need five pieces of paper. On the top of the first one write, "What did my parents and grandparents like to do? What were their passions?" Before we go any further, take a few minutes to answer that question and write down three to five or more things. For example, my grandfather on my dad's side was a carpenter, kind and observant. He loved games and was quite competitive. My mother used to speak of how upset he would be when I, even at the young age of seven, would beat him at checkers. My grandmother on dad's side would play dolls with me for hours and had always been a homemaker in her earlier years.

My father seemed to love learning and working. He held two jobs in the summers and usually brought work home in the evenings during the winter months. He loved words and writing and I recall his dragging out the dictionary at dinner (to my brother's and my chagrin at the time) to clarify some spelling or meaning of a word for us. He also was musically inclined and loved to sing and dance. I would often hear him singing in the morning as he prepared to go to work.

My grandmother on my mother's side died at age twenty-six of tuberculosis when my own mother was only a year and a half old. In her pictures, she looks like a beautiful woman who took great pride in her appearance. My mother's father was a farmer in Maine and died cutting wood in the forest when he was hit by a tree. I was very young and never met the man.

My mother was an extraordinary woman in her own right. She always put family first and had the cleanest house and best meals ever. She made our home a truly happy place, one that my friends all loved to visit. She did not drink and frowned on those who did. I suspect that that had something to do with her childhood, but I do not know for sure. Our home was "dry," so to speak, until my aunt would come for the holidays and needed to make the hard sauce for the plum pudding which apparently needed continual tasting in the making.

Mom was a Protestant, but did not practice in the church. It was my dad who took us to the Catholic church on Sundays, yet Mom would teach us the lessons in our catechisms. She converted to Catholicism later in life. She was industrious, often sewing our clothing and outfits for special occasions. She was thrifty and never wasted a thing.

Beyond being the leader in our family, Mom was also a leader outside the home, as president of the Parent Teacher's Association (PTA) and president of the Women's Club in town. She cared deeply about education and told my brother stories of working on the farm before running off to school as a small child, often being punished for showing up late, but never wanting to miss her studies.

The above are merely examples from my own life. Obviously, your sheet will look different from mine.

What Did You Love to Do as a Child?

On your second sheet, write the phrase, "Things I loved to do as a Child." Take a few minutes to list three to five things or more. Go back in time as far as you can. Again, by way of example, I was quite competitive as a child, especially enjoying games and mathematics. Growing up, I was often the "teacher's pet" in school. I was good at crochet and badminton, but never learned to swim and steered clear of most athletic activities. I loved social gatherings and arts and crafts.

Successes in Life

On the third sheet, write the words "Successes in Life" at the top. And yes, write down what you feel are your five or so most significant contributions, whether they be personal, school related, career related, health related, or whatever. Do not be modest. My own list includes staying married to the same guy for almost forty years now and raising our family of three kids, all of whom are contributing members of society and well educated; they each make us proud in so many ways. The list also includes holding executive positions in three diverse industries: telecom, energy services, and counseling. The last two of my five successes are earning the highest academic degree available and being financially independent, at least for now!

Attributes

Now, as you think about those successes in life, pick up a fourth sheet of paper and across the top write "Attributes." On this sheet, I want you to list the three to five or more skills or qualities you exhibited over time that allowed you to accomplish those successes. In case you need reminding, this is not a time to be modest. My list includes allegiance to commitments, leadership, organizing and planning, having a broad-based background, and being an incessant learner.

Future Imperatives

Take your last sheet and entitle it "Future Imperatives." Here, I want you to list as many things as you can, describing how you want your life to look going forward. Ask yourself how you can connect the things you loved as a child with your life today. Combine what you know about your ancestors and genes with experience and desires. Ask yourself, "What would make me feel fulfilled? What could help me grow? What would my ideal day and year look like? What would I be doing? Where would I be? What are my dreams?"

I have scripted such things as: commitment to family, learning from and influencing others, self development, becoming a spunky remarkable centenarian, and keeping my life in balance. Things that would make me feel fulfilled over time include staying healthy, writing and marketing my first book–and perhaps many others–teaching in some way, keeping up with technological and cultural changes, enjoying family and friends, and tracking finances to protect financial independence. Things that will assist in my growth will undoubtedly change over time but always be a work in process. This year, I am learning how to use Apple products such as the iPod, iPhone, and MacBook Air. I am still working on improving my tennis game, but as I learned in childhood, athletic activities are certainly not my strength. Still, all new learning counts.

My ideal day would find me close to family and friends sharing activities. My ideal year would encompass activities that ensure a balanced mix of intellectual, physical, social, emotional, and spiritual growth with fulfillment of specific goals such as walking 10,000 steps a day or publishing a book. My dream as a keen-ager is to replace the outdated image of "old people" as "old and unable" by setting a good example and inspiring others to do the same.

MY DREAM AS A KEEN-AGER IS TO REPLACE THE OUTDATED IMAGE OF "OLD PEOPLE" AS "OLD AND UNABLE" BY SETTING A GOOD EXAMPLE AND INSPIRING OTHERS TO DO THE SAME.

The Point of Intersection

Now put all your sheets in front of you. Is there anything you want to add? Are there any surprises or patterns that you see? My father loved learning and enjoyed writing. My grandmother on my mother's side seemed to take pride in her appearance. My mother was a leader in the family and community and cared deeply about education.

As you view the work you've done, you now want to pick out three or four elements and using your last sheet of paper, put the three or four elements selected in three or four circles, all of which intersect. That point where they intersect defines your sweet spot to the path forward. For example, in my case, I selected "learning from and influencing others," "becoming a spunky remarkable centenarian," and "writing and marketing my first book." My sweet spot is writing and marketing a book about midlife individuals becoming spunky remarkable centenarians and changing the image of "old people."

LEARNING FROM
AND INFLUENCING
OTHERS

BECOMING
A SPUNKY,
REMARKABLE
CENTENARIAN

SWEET
SPOT

WRITING AND
MARKETING MY
FIRST BOOK

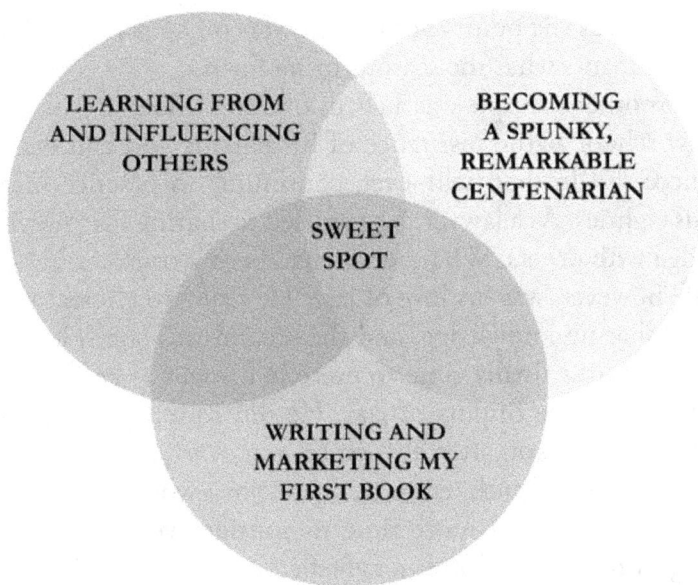

THE PATH FORWARD

Unfolding my complete package then, my sense of purpose (Who am I?) is to be the best I can be, help others be the best they can be, and in that way make the world a better place. My unique potential path (Who am I becoming?) is as an incessant learner focused on enriching longevity. And finally, my path forward is writing and marketing this book.

One of the women I know listed a pattern of her desires as reading, music, leadership, physical fitness, nature, travel, and talking. She had obtained a master gardener's degree. Selecting "leadership," "physical fitness," and "nature" for her circles, her point of introspection became clear. Now in her mid-seventies, she organizes and leads weekly hiking trips in the Carolinas. Her classes are so full, she sometimes has to limit registration. Her energy and passion shine through as she points out new flowers on a trail or shows participants what the seasons bring forth.

Another example was a client of mine who had gone to law school at the insistence of his parents and had been successful in that field–even continuing to practice into his eighties. As a lawyer, he was used to sharing his knowledge with others. What he said had been a constant in his life however, was his love of jazz. He had two circles; one was sharing knowledge, and the second was jazz. He decided it was finally time to exercise his wishes and teach classes on the origins of jazz. He did so and received a standing ovation after his first session.

The process outlined above is proven; it works. For those of you who need more time to consider your results, I highly recommend additional reflection on discoveries and any breakthroughs you might have had. Journaling and meditation can be useful resources for you. If you are a visual learner, you may benefit from performing the exercise utilizing pictures or objects. You may also want to revisit details in your background with relatives who are available to you.

The ideal outcome would be a new endeavor that thrills you. It may be something you have wanted to do for some time or something new you hadn't thought about until now. Either way, it must be consistent with your sense of purpose; you can see yourself getting up in the morning excited about the day and what follows. It is another step forward on your midlife leadership path whereby you are definitely practicing self leadership. Once engaged in the effort, you will know that it is exactly what you are supposed to be doing in your life right now. What could be better than that? You are on your path to unique potential.

SUMMARY AND CONCLUSION

"GROW OLD ALONG WITH ME
THE BEST IS YET TO BE. THE LAST OF LIFE,
FOR WHICH THE FIRST WAS MADE."
ROBERT BROWNING

Leadership in midlife is very much alive and well. We may no longer be leading others per se, but as keen-agers, we have the chance to lead ourselves in a direction that enriches our own lives as well as those around us. You're different, so why shouldn't your definition of effective leadership be different–but no less powerful?

Research and role models exist today to show us that becoming a remarkable centenarian, still full of life and focused on the future, or even a supercentenarian, is highly possible. We have developed a new vision detailing what that might look like for each of us.

In our earlier analogy, we learned that we will cycle through a "spiral of change," and I asked you to think about a corkscrew-like drilling process whereby you let go of something and take hold of something new with each turn. In the process of self discovery, we learned some new things about ourselves, and/or reinforced what we already knew. Keeping in mind a concept of "moderation," we looked at our life balance and regarded opportunities for new growth in the areas of intellectual stimulation, physical health, social networking, emotional literacy, and spiritual growth.

We then worked at crafting our sense of purpose to determine what fulfills us in life. Our final exercise and "uncorking" took us into the realm of our unique potential, that inner core that has been there all along, but may or may not have been tapped yet. Once tapped, we will have the information we need to capitalize on who we are and bring new excitement and growth into our lives. I am realizing my own unique potential by writing this book. It is clear to me that my own unique potential path is as "an incessant learner focused on enriching longevity."

Some of you will find yourselves totally "at home" with what you come up with, while others of you will want to consider that you have more learning to do. No direction you take is a mistake; it's all good and exactly where you are intended to be at that point. This is not an end point, but merely a stop along your journey in life. Do get started and get involved. There are no quick fixes here, but be sure that I will let you know if I find one. At this point, you are anointed a keen-ager and can consider yourselves fully launched, ready to take the steps necessary to move you towards your vision as an engaged centenarian. I hope you have enjoyed the journey so far, and I certainly encourage you to keep moving. Remember to keep in your circle of friends healthy people of all ages who share your forward thinking, positive outlook. They are the ones who will support you, bring you added joy, and celebrate your wins over the years. You will have the good fortune to do the same for them, and collectively, you will make the world a better place.

Come 2050, I look forward to a very large party, or maybe even a year of parties, to celebrate our collective wins and those yet ahead of us. Look for the notice of when and where. Or, maybe by then, we can just think about the location and time and know without reading it anywhere. Bring a present that represents your journey in some way, and we'll all exchange gifts. Don't have dessert the night before; there WILL be cake! Oh, and a glass of red wine for those who need their daily resveratrol. Expect lots of laughs and a chance to make new contacts in life. Our collective knowledge will be mind-boggling. I am also open to any parties before then for those of you who turn 100 or more before 2050; please invite me! Finally, you are all invited to my 120th birthday party in June 2065. Mark your calendars.

I will conclude with a favorite poem of mine by Linda Ellis. Some of you may have heard it before, but it is worth repeating. It's called "The Dash."

The Dash

At the funeral of his friend
He referred to the dates on her tombstone
From the beginning . . . to the end.

He noted that first came the date of her birth
And spoke of the second with tears,
But he said that what mattered most of all
Was the DASH between those years.

For that dash represents all the time
That she spent alive on earth,
And now only those who loved her
Know what that little line is worth . . .

Bibliography

Al-Anon Family Group Head Inc. Paths to Recovery: Al-Anon's Steps, Traditions, and Concepts. Virginia Beach: Al-Anon Family Group Head Inc., 1997.

Barnes, M. Craig. When God Interrupts: Finding New Life Through Unwanted Change. Downers Grove: InterVarsity Press, 1996.

Bellman, Geoffrey M. Your Signature Path: Gaining New Perspectives on Life. San Francisco: Berrett-Koehler Publishers, 1996.

Bennis, Warren. On Becoming a Leader. Cambridge: Perseus Books, 1994.

Buettner, Dan. The Blue Zones: Lessons for Living Longer From the People Who've Lived the Longest. Washington: National Geographic Society, 2008.

Bolman, Lee G., and Terrence E. Deal. Leading with Soul – An Uncommon Journey of Spirit. San Francisco: Jossey-Bass, 1995.

Cameron, Julia. The Artist's Way. New York: Penguin Putnam Inc., 1992.

Chilton, Floyd H. The Gene Smart Diet: The Revolutionary Eating Plan That Will Rewrite Your Genetic Destiny – And Melt Away the Pounds. With Laura Tucker. New York: Rodale Inc., 2009.

Corder, Roger. The Red Wine Diet. New York: The Penguin Group, 2007.

Covey, Stephen R. Principle-Centered Leadership. New York: Simon & Schuster Inc., 1992.

Covey, Stephen R., A. Roger Merrill, and Rebecca R. Merrill. First Things First: to Live, to Love, to Learn, to Leave a Legacy. New York: Simon & Schuster, 1994.

Crowley, Chris, and Henry S. Lodge. Younger Next Year: Live Strong, Fit, and Sexy – Until You're 80 and Beyond. New York: Workman Publishing, 2004.

Davidson, Sara. Leap!: What Will We Do with the Rest of Our Lives? New York: Random House, Inc., 2007.

Gauld, Joseph W. Character First: The Hyde School Way and Why It Works. San Francisco: Institute for Contemporary Studies Press, 1993.

Gertz, Dwight L., and Joao P. A. Baptista. Grow to be Great: Breaking the Downsizing Cycle. New York: The Free Press, 1995.

Gilbert, Daniel. Stumbling on Happiness. New York: Random House, Inc., 2005.

Goleman, Daniel. Social Intelligence: Why It Can Matter More Than IQ. New York: Random House, Inc., 2006.

Hanh, Thich Nhat, Arnold Kotler, and H. H. the Dalai

Lama. Peace Is Every Step – The Path of Mindfulness in Everyday Life. New York: Bantam Books, 1991.

Hudson, Frederic M. The Adult Years: Mastering the Art of Self-Renewal. San Francisco: Jossey-Bass, 1999.

Jaworski, Joseph. Synchronicity: The Inner Path of Leadership. San Francisco: Berrett-Koehler Publishers, 1996.

Jeffers, Susan. Feel the Fear . . . and Do It Anyway. New York: Ballantine Books, 1987.

Jones, Laurie Beth. Jesus, CEO: Using Ancient Wisdom for Visionary Leadership. New York: Hyperion, 1995.

Jung, C.G., edited by Campbell, Joseph. The Portable Jung. (pp. 178-269). New York: Penguin Books, 1976.

Kundera, Milan. The Book of Laughter and Forgetting. trans. Michael Henry Heim. New York: Alfred A. Knopf, Inc., 1980.

Levinson, Daniel J. The Seasons of a Man's Life. New York: Ballantine Books, 1978.

Maffetone, Philip. In Fitness and In Health. 3rd ed. Stamford: David Barmore Productions, 1997.

McLean, Pamela D., and Frederic M. Hudson. LifeLaunch – A Passionate Guide to the Rest of Your Life. Santa Barbara: the Hudson Institute Press, 1996.

Moore, Thomas. Care of the Soul: A Guide for Cultivating Depth and Sacredness in Everyday Life. New York: Harper Perennial, 1992.

Myers, I. B., & McCaulley, M. H. Manual: A Guide to the Development and the Use of the Myers-Briggs Type Indicator. Palo Alto, CA: Consulting Psychologists Press, 1985.

O'Neil, John R. The Paradox of Success. New York: G.P. Putnam's Sons, 1994.

Perls, Thomas T., and Margery Hutter Silver. Living to 100: Lessons in Living to Your Maximum Potential at Any Age. New York: Basic Books, 1999.

Phillips, Bob. Over the Hill and Still Rolling: Jolly Jokes for (Not So) Older Folks. Eugene: Harvest House Publishers, 2001.

Quinn, Robert E. Deep Change: Discovering the Leader Within. San Francisco: Jossey-Bass, 1996.

Rogers, Carl R. On Becoming a Person: A Therapist's View of Psychotherapy. New York: Houghton Mifflin Company, 1995.

Sanborn, Mark. You Don't Need a Title to Be a Leader. Random House audio tapes, 2006.

Schneider, Edward L., and Elizabeth Miles. AgeLess: Take Control of Your Age and Stay Youthful for Life. New York: St. Martin's Press, 2003.

Sheehy, Gail. The Silent Passage. New York: Pocket Books, 1991.

Sheehy, Gail. New Passages: Mapping Your Life Across Time. New York: Ballantine Books, 1995.

Sher, Barbara. I Could Do Anything If I Only Knew What It Was. With Barbara Smith. New York: Dell Publishing, 1994.

Vaill, Peter B. Learning as a Way of Being: Strategies for Survival in a World of Permanent White Water. San Francisco: Jossey-Bass, 1996.

Vaillant, George E. Aging Well: Surprising Guideposts to a Happier Life. New York: Little Brown and Company, 2002.

Ward-Baker, Patricia D. "The Remarkable Oldest Old: A New Vision of Aging." Ph.D. diss. University of Michigan, 2006. ProQuest Publication Number 3228133.

Werner, Carrie A. "The Older Population." Washington: Census Briefs, 2011.

ABOUT THE AUTHOR

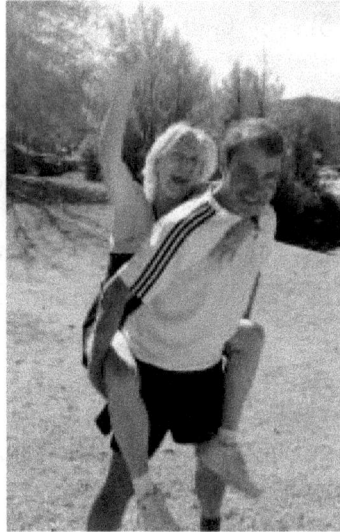

Dr. Tricia Keene is the proud mother of three young adults, and wife of Warren for 39 years–and counting. She spent 30 years working in the telecommunications and energy services industries, up to and including the executive level.

At age 56, she earned her Ph.D. with a concentration in midlife leadership, while working as an executive, counseling clients worldwide who were going through life transitions. Since then, she has worked with clients and taught numerous classes to hundreds of participants in their late 40s to mid 90s. She is an incessant learner focused on enriching longevity.

Dr. Keene, in her bid to have readers live their best lives– to age 120 or beyond–capitalizes on concepts based in years of experience, research and interviews. She believes that setting a positive long-term goal for aging matters, and she lives the life her research has deemed the best path to get there. Dr. Keene intends to change the image of "senior" adults from one of "old and unable" to one of "vibrant and valuable."

You may contact Dr. Keene at Tricia@Enjoyto120.com, or visit her website Enjoyto120.com.